A Beginner's Guide to Evidence-Based Practice in Health and Social Care

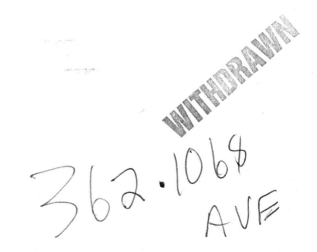

A Beginner's Guide to Evidence-Based Practice in Health and Social Care

Second Edition

Helen Aveyard and Pam Sharp

 Open University Press

Open University Press
McGraw-Hill Education
McGraw-Hill House
Shoppenhangers Road
Maidenhead
Berkshire
England
SL6 2QL

email: enquiries@openup.co.uk
world wide web: www.openup.co.uk

and Two Penn Plaza, New York, NY 10121-2289, USA

First published 2009
Reprinted 2010, 2011 (twice), 2012
First published in this second edition 2013

Copyright © Helen Aveyard & Pam Sharp, 2013

A catalogue record of this book is available from the British Library

ISBN-13: 978-0-335-24672-4
ISBN-10: 0-335-24672-9
eISBN: 978-0-335-24673-1

Library of Congress Cataloging-in-Publication Data
CIP data applied for

Typeset by Aptara, Inc.
Printed and bound by CPI Group (UK) Ltd, Croydon, CR0 4YY

Fictitious names of companies, products, people, characters and/or data that may
be used herein (in case studies or in examples) are not intended to represent any
real individual, company, product or event.

Praise for this book

"The jargon-free accessible language and up-to-date examples and links in this book will make it a valuable resource for a range of health professionals as well as for those teaching them. The importance of EBP means that this text will be relevant for experienced practitioners as much as for students embarking on a career in health and social care."
Sally Dowling, Senior Lecturer, Adult Nursing, University of the West of England, UK

"This is a book that I recommend without reservation, and one that despite the title will be helpful to those who are not beginners. It is written clearly without being patronizing. The activities help relate it to practice. Whether it is for an assignment or to change practice, this book will help you obtain the relevant evidence, appraise it and demonstrate that it is convincing and useful in relation to your work place."
Patric Devitt, Senior Lecturer, School of Nursing, Midwifery & Social Work, University of Salford, UK

"Even as a Third Year Nursing Degree student this book has been a lifesaver."
Amazon review

Contents

Acknowledgements

We would like to thank the following individuals for their help during the writing of this book.

Jill Gregory for proof reading the manuscript

Tim Sharp for his support and patience. Dave, Zack and Adam Stubbs for their welcome distraction

Paul, Benedict and Edward Aveyard for being there

Introduction

This book is for you if you are:

- A student starting out or undertaking a pre-registration course in any of the health and social care professions.
- A registered practitioner, who may be returning to post-qualification study or to practice after a career break.
- Anyone who feels clinically or professionally 'out of date' or has ever said '*I am not an academic . . . I am practical*' or '*I've always done it this way*'.
- A practice assessor/mentor[1] who is supporting students in practice and aware of the need to use evidence in your daily practice and to role model best practice to your students.

This book is for you if you already know that:

- You are legally and professionally accountable for your practice once you are a registered practitioner.
- As a student you may be called to account by your university or institution of higher education.
- There is a large amount and many different types of information available.
- You need skills in order to find, understand and use information.
- In order to function safely and/or to be successful as a student (pre- or post-qualifying) or member of staff you need to know how to apply relevant information to your practice and in your written work.

So . . . where do you start?
You might feel that you do not know where to begin to use this evidence in your practice and learning or that when you try to it is too complicated or

---

[1] The term practice assessor/mentor will be used throughout to describe those who support learners in practice. A variety of terms are used throughout the professions such as: clinical educator, supervisor, practice educator/teacher, clinical tutor or instructor.

difficult. This book will lead you through this process at an introductory level in a jargon-free way.

Aim of this book

The aim of this book is to explain evidence-based practice (EBP) and to present it as a topic that practitioners of all levels, including students, can relate to from the very start of their professional experience and in their writing. Evidence-based practice is of course a practical topic; however, we are aware that it is assessed in academic writing and is a substantial component in almost all marking criteria for those studying for a professional qualification in health and social care.

A Beginner's Guide to Evidence-Based Practice in Health and Social Care provides a step-by-step approach to using evidence in practice in a practical and straightforward way.

Examples

We have tried to include examples that may be generally understood and by a range of professions as we all work within a wider team. We would ask that you read through the examples even if they don't relate directly to your profession and think broadly about the message the example is giving.

How to get the most from this book

- Try and read the introductory chapters first as the book is presented in the order we think it should be read, but you can use the index if you have a particular issue you want to find out about.
- Use the glossary for explanations of words you are unfamiliar with.
- Work with a colleague or a student who is more confident in using evidence in practice.
- Get access to the internet and start practising 'searching' using relevant databases (don't leave it until you really need to find information quickly).
- Do some additional reading around the topic of EBP.
- Contact your local health and social care librarian (through your work organization or local university) for additional, practical training sessions. Some university libraries have specialist health and social care librarians.
- Don't give up if you find something difficult or don't understand it. Feel good about every new thing that you have learnt.

Use the symbols

Key information

Think point

Activity for you to do

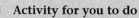

1

What is evidence-based practice?

Have clear reasons for your practice decisions and your care • Defining evidence-based practice • Exploring the components of evidence-based practice • Consequences of not taking an evidence-based approach • What does evidence-based practice mean to me? • In summary • Key points

 Simply put, EBP is practice that is supported by a clear, up-to-date rationale, taking into account the patient/client's preferences and using your own judgement. If we practise an evidence-based approach then we are set to give the best possible care.

Sounds complicated? It's not really, just read on...
Evidence-based practice starts with the following principle:

Have clear reasons for your practice decisions and your care

If you are a **student** starting out on a course in any of the health and social care professions, you are likely to be well aware of the need to be able to explain the care that you give both in practice and in the assignments you write. This is because patients and clients expect you, even as a student, to understand why you are caring for them in a particular way and to explain the reasons (or **rationale**) for the care you give. This becomes increasingly important as you gain experience and become the one who is planning care and making decisions relating to care, rather than acting in a more supportive role. In fact, being able to explain a good rationale for our practice decisions and planning care is one of the things that distinguishes registered health and social care practitioners from those in assistant roles.

As a **registered practitioner** you may feel that you cannot always give a thorough rationale for your practice, and fear that your practice may not be as up-to-date as it could be, and this can make you feel vulnerable or under-confident. You may not have been able to access professional development opportunities or you may be about to re-start study and want to find out how to use evidence in your academic work.

If you are a **practice assessor/mentor** supervising learners or a **practitioner** who is returning to work or study after a career break, you are likely to be even more aware of this need. You may feel lacking in skills to act as a role model for best practice and lack confidence in giving reasons for your practice to others. Consider the following examples:

Examples from practice

Example 1: Imagine you are a social work student. Your current placement is with a multidisciplinary team which works in a deprived area of the country. The case load includes a lot of disadvantaged families. You visit one family in which one of the members, a 5-year-old child, has behavioural problems. The family are given advice about attending a parenting skills programme for help in managing the behaviour of the child. When you leave the family home, you ask your practice assessor/mentor why this has been advised. They explain that support provided by parenting groups can help the parents to manage the behaviour of their child and to relieve their own stress and anxiety caused by the child's difficulties.

Example 2: Imagine you are a health visitor working in an immunization clinic. Although the health scare surrounding the MMR vaccinations has largely diminished, there are still many parents who want to know what the scare was about and whether it has been truly resolved. On one occasion you find that you have to give very specific information to allay the fears of a young mother. After you have provided a detailed rationale for why the vaccination is now considered safe, and why you are happy to give it, the mother appears reassured and agrees to the vaccination for her child.

Example 3: Now imagine you are working in a travel vaccination clinic and are consulted by a patient who is travelling far afield on a gap year. The patient asks you in a lot of detail for information about the risks and benefits of various vaccinations and you do not feel confident to answer her questions. In fact, some of her questions remind you that you are not as fully aware of

---

the rationale for the advice given as you might be. You resort to statements such as 'This is what we always give to people going to that area . . .' but you can sense that the patient is keen to know more to ensure that she is fully protected and to consider any alternative courses of action that might be available to her, including altering her travel plans. If you were the patient attending the clinic, how confident would you be about the advice offered if the practitioner was not able to give you a clear rationale?

You can see from these simple examples that as a student or registered member of staff, it is essential that you can provide a clear rationale for the care you give. You need to be able to tell the patient/client/student why an intervention or procedure is required and be able to provide a clear rationale. This is part of EBP.

But providing a rationale alone is not enough

Being able to provide a clear rationale for the care you give is essential but not quite sufficient.

 An EBP approach requires that we ensure our rationale is not only *clear* but also *up to date and based on the best available evidence.*

In other words you need to be able to defend your practice and ensure that you have a good rationale for the actions you have taken. Wherever possible your rationale should be based on the **best possible evidence** although what we mean by 'evidence' is very broadly defined and is different in different cases. There are **lots of different types of evidence** that we can draw on to underpin practice and we will discuss these throughout this book. Often the best evidence will be research studies or, better still a review of all research studies undertaken in an area. Let's look back to the example about the social work student on placement and the advice given to the family with the child with the behavioural problems. The multidisciplinary team knew about the provision of groups that might help the parents cope with the behaviour of the child. However this alone is not enough. Where public resources and services may be limited, we need to be as sure as we can that the support groups are likely to be useful and effective if they are to be provided for parents. We need to be aware of the **evidence** or **rationale** for the care we provide and to be sure that the evidence or rationale is **robust.** In this case, the social worker explained her rationale to the student. This rationale is based on a large review of many different research studies which had evaluated the impact of parenting groups for children with behavioural difficulties

(Furlong *et al.* 2012). The conclusion of this review was that the provision of parenting classes was beneficial to both the subsequent behaviour of the child and the stress and anxiety of the family unit.

Defining evidence-based practice

Evidence-based practice is not just about evidence. David Sackett, founder of the NHS Research and Development Centre for Evidence-Based Medicine in Oxford, and colleagues defined EBP as follows:

Evidence-based practice is: 'The conscientious and judicious use of current best evidence in conjunction with clinical expertise and patient values to guide health [*and social*] care decisions'. (Sackett *et al.* 2000: 71–72)

Sackett and colleagues emphasize that there is a strong link between EBP and the decisions we make in our everyday practice. Our decisions should be clearly stated and well-thought through (judicious), and use evidence sensibly and carefully. They also emphasize the role of **professional judgement** and **patient or client preference** within the idea of EBP. That is, they argue, evidence alone is not enough; it should be supplemented with the judgement of the practitioner and the wishes of the patient or client.

Dawes *et al.* (2005: 7) in the Sicily statement offer a similar, yet more holistic definition of EBP. They emphasize the role of evidence in addition to the tacit and explicit knowledge of the care givers and the views of the patient or client.

Evidence Based Practice (EBP) requires that decisions about health and social care are based on the best available, current, valid and relevant evidence. These decisions should be made by those receiving care, informed by the tacit and explicit knowledge of those providing care, within the context of available resources.

In order to emphasize the role of professional judgement and to counteract the misunderstandings that *evidence-based practice* was just about research and that it did not value the judgement of the practitioner and the patient's own views, the term *'evidence-informed practice'* has emerged. This seems to be a more acceptable term for those involved in complementary and alternative medicine and those involved in work that involves interventions with more human contact and communication. Nevo and Slomin-Nevo (2011: 1) refer to the term **evidence-informed practice** (EIP) and argue that the principles of evidence and professional judgement should be central to our approach to patient or client care. So they think **evidence-informed practice** should be understood as:

> excluding non-scientific prejudices and superstitions, but also as leaving ample room for clinical experience as well as the constructive and imaginative judgements of practitioners and clients who are in constant interaction and dialogue with one another.

 Where do you think the balance should lie between the health and social care provider making a decision and that decision being made by those in receipt of care?

Different terminology used

We have defined EBP as we understand it. However there are many different terms that refer to the broader concept of 'evidence-based practice' or 'evidence-informed practice'. These are amongst others:

- Evidence-Based Medicine
- Research-Based Practice
- Evidence-Based Nursing
- Evidence-Based Physiotherapy
- Evidence-Based Dietetics
- Evidence-Based Midwifery
- Evidence-Based Occupational Therapy.

If you were to study the exact components of each you might find slight variations in emphasis in the definitions but you would find general agreement that all definitions include **use of evidence** combined with **professional opinion and patient or client preference.** We would argue that despite differences in nuance, these terms share the same overriding philosophy and are discussed below.

Arguably, there is one approach that falls slightly outside our definitions and is referred to as 'values-based practice'. Fulford (2010) describes the role of **values-based practice** as a partner to EBP, the role of which is to balance decision making within health and social care within a framework of shared values. It is beyond the scope of this book to explore this idea in detail, however there are many similarities between the approaches of 'evidence-based practice' and 'values-based practice'. Given that professional opinion, patient or client preference and the use of evidence are central to the concept of EBP and VBP, it could be argued that the two frameworks are not dissimilar. Again this is a question of nuance, rather than a parallel or competing framework.

Exploring the components of evidence-based practice

The main definitions of EBP agree that there are three main components:

- Use of evidence.
- Clinical or professional judgement.
- Patient/client preference.

We will now look at each of these ideas in turn:

Use of evidence

We have discussed in earlier examples how evidence has been used by practitioners to justify the rationale for the care they give and how evidence is a central component of EBP. We need evidence and it must be good evidence. In Chapter 6 we will discuss how you can tell if the evidence is strong or not. What has changed in recent years is the acknowledgement that the term 'evidence' is quite broad and you could be looking at many diverse sources of evidence and other information to justify your practice. We will discuss the type of evidence you might come across in detail in Chapter 4 but in summary, the term 'evidence' does not just refer to research done in a lab under strict controlled conditions! The best evidence for our professional practice is usually some type of research evidence if it is available.

Consider how you would value the findings of a well-conducted piece of research that compared different ways of quitting smoking to an anecdotal account from one person who had tried to quit and had failed to do so.

You can usually recognize a piece of research by the way it is presented. Research is usually written up in a paper published in one of the professional journals. Professional journals, such as *Journal of Advanced Nursing* or *Addiction* are often considered to be the gold standard of professional information because the material has always been **peer reviewed** and checked before accepted for publication. A research study usually starts with a question – called the research question – which the researchers then seek to answer by a method which is clearly stated in the research paper, followed by the results and then discussion of what these results are likely to mean.

In an ideal situation, we would use not just one research study, but a review of studies (sometimes called a literature review or a **systematic review**). A review of evidence provides stronger evidence than a single study because identifying the whole range of studies about a topic is more reliable than the results of just one, which might be misleading or provide an inaccurate picture.

The study referred to earlier by Furlong *et al.* (2012) is an example of a systematic review. The term 'systematic' refers to a review of the literature or evidence that has been carried out in a systematic and rigorous way and such reviews are generally high quality evidence. The most well-known systematic reviews are those produced by **the Cochrane** or **Campbell Collaboration** which we will refer to later on in this book.

If you come across a review published by either the Cochrane or Campbell Collaborations, then you have probably come across good quality evidence.

If there are no systematic reviews or literature reviews on the topic you are interested in, then the next best thing is to find a research study or several studies on your topic. *The types of study you are looking for will depend on the focus or question you are trying to address* and we will discuss this in Chapter 4. There are many different approaches to research and we will consider these later. It is important to emphasize that different types of research are needed for different types of situations. It is not helpful to say that one type of research is 'better' than another – it all depends on the aim of the research. It is however possible and necessary to make a judgement about the quality of the research and whether it has been well done or not – and we will discuss how to do this in Chapter 6.

It may sometimes be the case that there is **not sufficient research evidence** upon which to base practice or you find that the research evidence is **inconclusive** or of **poor quality.** There might be a lack of evidence because it is unethical to undertake research to explore the particular area you are interested in. It may also be the case that there is research but it **does not directly apply** to your particular area and you need to use your **professional judgement** as to whether the research can be applied in the context in which you are working. There will also be times when you need to draw on alternative sources of evidence other than research evidence alone.

However, it is important to note that it is **research** that often – but not always – provides the strongest **evidence** upon which we base our practice and is at the heart of EBP. However research evidence alone is not enough for your practice. This is why the definitions of EBP include referring to your professional judgement and patient or client preference. We will now address this component of EBP.

Evidence-based practice and clinical/professional judgement and intuition

There is sometimes an incorrect assumption that EBP refers to the use of research alone. You might hear people say '*evidence-based practice is too rigid and doesn't relate to real experiences*'.

As we have already mentioned, evidence alone is not enough for EBP. Our own professional or clinical judgement is vital for assisting with providing an evidence-based approach to care. In their early discussion of EBP, Sackett and colleagues (1996) describe how evidence can inform decisions about practice, but cannot replace professional expertise and judgement. They argue that this clinical/professional expertise is used to determine whether the available evidence should be applied to the individual patient/client at all and, if so, if it should be used to inform our decision making.

It is important that all the evidence we use is professionally evaluated, because every patient or client context is unique. Tanner (2006: 204) defined clinical (or professional) judgement as:

> an interpretation or conclusion about a patient's needs, concerns, or health problems, and/or the decision to take action (or not), use or modify standard approaches, or improvise new ones as deemed appropriate by the patient's response.

This definition recognizes the *patients' preferences* as part of EBP and Downie and Macnaughten (2009) further describe professional judgement as 'an assertion made with *evidence or good reason* in a context of uncertainty' (p. 322).

Professional or clinical judgement may also be used alongside intuition. Intuition is often referred to as gut feeling '(just knowing)'.

- There appears to be a close relationship between experience and intuition.
- Intuition is grounded in both knowledge and experience in making judgements.

(Benner 1984; Benner and Tanner 1987)

Intuition can be incorporated into EBP when clinical or professional judgement is applied. Indeed this was argued by Benner and Tanner back in 1987 who described how intuitive knowledge and analytical reasoning are not opposed to each other – they can and do work together.

Professional judgement can also be important if there is not sufficient evidence, or the evidence does not refer to the specific patient/client we are looking after. Therefore a judgement is needed as to the relevance of the evidence we have to the particular **context, complexity** and the **individuality** of patient or client.

Where there is no reliable research evidence, the judgement of the practitioner *IS* the best evidence.

What evidence is there to support using intuition?

The importance of professional judgement and intuition was reinforced in a literature review (McGraughey *et al.* 2009) which gathered together the evidence about the use of checklists versus professional judgement/intuition in the nursing assessment of patients whose condition had rapidly deteriorated. The use of checklists to trigger nursing staff to refer a patient for urgent medical attention has become widely used. They are promoted as a way of standardizing the referral for urgent medical attention and, in theory at least, replace the nurses' intuition with a more objective approach. This is in addition to the interpretation of the patient's vital signs which checks whether or not the patient's condition has deteriorated. The question of whether the use of these checklists has made hospital a safer place for patients whose condition deteriorates has been researched in various studies. And so, McGraughey and colleagues (2009) carried out a systematic review and compared the results of all of these studies. In their review, they found that nurses' intuition was as reliable a trigger for seeking medical help as the use of a checklist or tool. This is maybe why some health and social care practitioners state that their **professional work is an art as well as a science** and it incorporates a human element which cannot be reduced to just the application of research knowledge to patient/client care. This can be described as clinical or professional judgement.

It is important to emphasize that intuition and experience are used in conjunction with an evidence-based approach,

 Using evidence without professional judgement can lead to formulaic care and using professional judgement without available evidence can lead to the perpetuation of outdated practice. The two should work together!

So far, we have argued that EBP requires more than 'raw' evidence. It requires clinical or professional judgement. This may be based on intuition and/or experience so that the evidence can be appropriately applied in practice. Now let's look at patient/client preferences and what role they play in EBP.

Evidence-based practice and patient/client preference

There is also a third component – that the patient/client's preference must be acknowledged and their **consent** sought prior to the undertaking of any intervention. If all the best evidence and clinical or professional judgement pointed towards an intervention or therapy that the patient/client did not accept, then we should not carry it out.

Find out what your professional body says about consent prior to undertaking care, or interventions.

All care delivered must be with the agreement or consent of the patient/client. Not only does the patient have a legal right to make his or her own decisions (in most countries) but in addition, there has been recent debate about the importance of shared decision making and increased patient/client involvement in the health and social care context. In the UK, this is reflected in the Department of Health (2012) consultation document entitled *Liberating the NHS – No Decision About Me Without Me,* which emphasizes the importance of the role of the patient or client in decision making. The consultation document is about the need to involve the public in care decisions and make information available to them in accessible formats. The document asserts that the NHS will put patients at the heart of the NHS, through an information revolution and greater choice and control, with an emphasis on shared decision making and patient access to information. (This consultation paper is available at: http://www.dh.gov.uk/prod_consum_dh/groups/dh_ digitalassets/@dh/@en/documents/digitalasset/dh_134218.pdf).

These principles are also grounded in law. In legal terms, any care that is delivered without the patient/client's consent may be unlawful. The exception to this is if the patient is temporarily (in an emergency) or permanently unable to consent. In these cases, care for patient/clients should be delivered that is in their best interests. Care for those who are unable to consent is determined in The Mental Capacity Act (Department of Constitutional Affairs 2005, implemented 2007, available at http://www.legislation.gov.uk/ukpga/2005/9/contents).

The Mental Capacity Act:

- Presumes capacity
- Reinforces the right of individuals to be supported to make decisions
- Reinforces the right of individuals to make eccentric or unwise decisions
- Reinforces that anything done for or on behalf of people without capacity must be done 'in their best interests'
- Reinforces that anything done for or on behalf of people without capacity should be least restrictive of rights and freedoms.

Check that you are fully aware of the principles regarding informed consent.

There is some evidence to suggest that urgent care is sometimes delayed because practitioners are not aware that they can deliver care that is in the best interests of a patient or client who cannot consent (Variend 2012).

Some patient/clients really want to be involved in the decisions relating to their care. Others will want to trust that the practitioner will make the best possible decision on their behalf. This is a big responsibility and we need to be well informed as to what might be the best option for our patient/clients. There are decision aids available to help patients who need to make treatment choices on the NHS direct website (http://www.nhsdirect.nhs.uk/decisionaids).

The main point to remember is that the care cannot be delivered without the consent of the patient/client and if you do not gain consent as a practitioner, you are at risk of professional misconduct and in breach of the law unless the patient or client lacks the ability to consent.

What are the consequences of not taking an evidence-based approach?

Although delivery of the **best possible care** is the main driver behind EBP, there are consequences for you as a practitioner if you are not able to explain your care decisions and these will now be discussed.

Example from practice

Imagine you are the patient attending the travel clinic referred to earlier. You want to seek advice about the vaccinations required before you go abroad on a tropical holiday. Unfortunately, the practitioner is not up to date with current practice and recommends a vaccine which is now rarely used and has been largely replaced by a newer vaccine which has been found, due to large scale research studies, to be far more effective. The practitioner has been administering this older vaccine for years and is unaware of the newer more effective vaccination. They are therefore not practising EBP because they are not using the best up-to-date evidence to inform their practice.

Meanwhile your friend, who is travelling with you, visits a different practitioner and is given the new vaccine. You experience some unpleasant side effects and when you read up about the vaccine, you discover that your friend is better protected than you are against the disease in question – and did not experience any side effects! You feel angry and your trust in the practitioner who had not given you the most up-to-date and best available healthcare is broken.

Accountability

In the example above, you might feel like making a complaint against the practitioner who gave you the out-of-date vaccine, especially if it caused you to have unpleasant side effects or reduced your enjoyment of the holiday because you feared that you were not fully protected by the vaccination. If you did make a complaint, the practitioner would then have to justify why this out-of-date vaccine was given. This would be difficult to do if all the evidence pointed towards the newer vaccine.

As a health or social care practitioner, you are *accountable* to your manager or university (if you are a student), your professional organization and to the law.

This means that you must be able to justify and give a clear account of and rationale for your practice. Failure to do this can result in professional misconduct.

- Students are accountable to their higher education institution and when in practice should be supervised by a registered practitioner.
- Registered practitioners are accountable to their professional body and their employers.
- We are all accountable to the law.

If there was a standard or policy document in his or her place of work that recommended the newer vaccine, then the practitioner would find it difficult to justify administering the old vaccine. Even if no such documentation existed, the practitioner would still find it difficult to justify why an outdated vaccine was administered when a more effective vaccine with fewer side effects was available.

We can see that when you are called to account for your practice, you will only be able to do so if you have administered care that is based on the best available evidence. You will not be able to account for care that is based on old or weak evidence.

Find out what your *professional body, college* or *association* says about your accountability and evidence-based practice.

In the United Kingdom these are as follows:

For **allied health professions and social workers** including: occupational therapists, physiotherapists, operating department practitioners, dieticians, paramedics, radiographers, speech and language therapists, art therapists, chiropodists/podiatrists, clinical scientists, orthoptists, prosthetists and orthotists the **Health and Care Professions Council** (HCPC). They publish their Standards of Conduct, Performance and Ethics (2012) (available at: http://www.hpc-uk.org/aboutregistration/standards/).

They state that 'you must keep your professional knowledge and skills up to date' (HCPC 2012:10).

For nurses: the **Nursing and Midwifery Council (NMC)**. They publish The Code, their Standards of Conduct, Performance and Ethics (2008) (available at http://www.nmc-uk.org/Publications/Standards/The-code/Introduction/).

The Code requires all practitioners to deliver evidence-based care. Practitioners are required to 'deliver care based on the **best available evidence** or best practice' (NMC 2008: 7). The Code declares that nurses and midwives are **accountable** for the care they deliver.

Therefore, if you are called upon to account for your practice, you must be able to provide a sound rationale for why you acted as you did. If you are only able to say '*I was told to do this*' or '*I've always done it this way*', your practice will look very poor indeed! Students are expected to work towards these standards in order to obtain registration and failure to do so may affect progression towards qualification.

Individual colleges or associations may also be involved in setting professional guidance and you should access their websites to see what relates to your own profession.

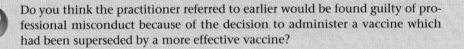

Do you think the practitioner referred to earlier would be found guilty of professional misconduct because of the decision to administer a vaccine which had been superseded by a more effective vaccine?

Would that verdict have been reached if he/she had used an evidence-based approach to the selection of the appropriate vaccine?

Clinical governance

In addition to accountability through the professional governing bodies, in the UK, health and social care practitioners are also accountable to the organization in which they work through the concept of clinical governance. Whilst the mechanisms of clinical governance are liable to change, the concept of clinical governance is that of accountability of the individual practitioner to the institution in which he or she is employed (http://www.dh.gov.uk/health/2011/09/clinical-governance/).

The purpose of clinical governance is to ensure that the institution – in addition to the individual practitioner – is accountable for the care that its service provides.

The government website (http://www.dh.gov.uk/health/2011/09/clinical-governance/) on clinical governance explains that:

Clinical governance' describes the structures, processes and culture needed to ensure that healthcare organisations – and all individuals within them – can assure the quality of the care they provide and are continuously seeking to improve it.

The Kings Fund offers a directory of the monitoring and quality organizations including the Quality Care Commission (http://www.kingsfund.org.uk/topics/governance_regulation_and_accountability/index.html).

Part of this governance is ensuring staff are educated and trained and that they are using up-to-date interventions.

In addition, the **Essence of Care** benchmarking statements have been designed to contribute to the introduction of clinical governance at local level. The benchmarking process outlined in 'The essence of care' statements 'helps practitioners to take a structured approach to sharing and comparing practice, enabling them to identify the **best practice** and to develop action plans to remedy poor practice' (DH 2010). (These documents are available at: http://www.dh.gov.uk/en/Publication sandstatistics/Publications/PublicationsPolicyAndGuidance/DH_119969).

Standards and quality assurance initiatives will be present in **non-NHS organizations** too.

Legal considerations

Finally, in addition to accountability to the relevant professional body and employing institution, as registered practitioners you are accountable to the law. The main area of law in the UK that is likely to be of relevance to those working within health and social care is the tort of negligence. Being able to justify the care that you give may protect you or your organization from a claim in negligence. There is a developing culture of litigation and claims against health and social care organizations. Patients or clients who are unhappy about the care they receive can make a claim in negligence if they have suffered harm as a result of that care. There is a National Health Service Litigation Authority (NHSLA, http://www.nhsla.com/home.htm) that handles negligence claims and works to improve risk management practices in the NHS. Clinical governance, discussed earlier, includes several measures to ensure we provide safe and effective care.

Let's return to the **example** about the administration of an outdated travel vaccination. Let's say that the worst does happen and you contract a serious tropical disease whilst you are away, the disease against which you had been vaccinated (with the less effective vaccine). Your travelling companion does not contract the disease. You become very ill and lose sight in one eye and are unable to work. In order to seek compensation you make a claim of negligence against the healthcare provider who did not use the best available evidence when selecting your travel vaccinations.

To make a successful claim in negligence against a health and social care provider, the patient/client has to demonstrate that the healthcare provider failed in their duty to provide care and that this failure led to harm. The courts have consistently ruled that such a failure occurs if the health or social care provider has provided care that is not evidence based. In this case, the administration of an outdated vaccine that is less effective than its newer version led to a greater likelihood of your contracting the disease and might lead to a claim of negligence. Under the current system, you can only make a claim in negligence if you have suffered harm. Therefore, you would not be able to claim in negligence just because you had received the less effective vaccine; you would only be able to make a claim if you did contract the disease or suffered some other harm.

Let's then say that unfortunately your friend also contracts the disease, despite receiving the newer vaccine – (no vaccination is ever 100 per cent effective). If (s)he then attempts to bring a case in negligence against the health and social care provider, (s)he is less likely to be able to succeed because the practitioner in this case used the most up-to-date evidence to select the appropriate vaccine and hence did not fail in the duty owed to the patient/client.

Being able to provide a good rationale or explanation for your practice is an essential component of the concept 'evidence-based practice' and might even prevent you from becoming involved in any legal proceedings.

Therefore, you can see that you are less likely to make errors or give the wrong information to your service users if you follow recommendations for best practice and have a sound rationale for what you do.

What does evidence-based practice mean to me?

So far in this chapter we have introduced the concept of EBP and why we feel it is so important. We have used examples from professional health and social care practice to illustrate this and the likely implications that can arise from following a 'non evidence-based' approach.

Throughout this book, we will look in more detail at how you might achieve an evidence-based approach. The following approach (adapted from Thompson *et al.* 2005) provides an illustration of how an evidence-based approach may be used in professional practice and we identify where in this book we discuss the stages of using an evidence-based approach.

1 **Identify what you need to find out:** this may be information or evidence about the best care for an individual patient or client or at a wider public health level. In this chapter we have identified examples where

practitioners needed to find specific evidence to enable them to provide the best 'evidence-based care'.

2 **Search for the most appropriate evidence:** this is usually research evidence but could be other forms of evidence as we will discuss in Chapter 5.

3 **Try to work out if the evidence you find is any good:** we refer to this process as 'critical appraisal of the evidence' and we will discuss how we assess evidence in Chapter 6.

4 **Incorporate the evidence into a strategy for action:** if the evidence is good enough, remember to refer to your professional judgement and patient or client preference. We will discuss this further in Chapter 7.

5 **Evaluate the effects of any decisions and action taken:** this will be discussed further in Chapter 7.

Examples from practice

Example 1: Let's imagine you have noticed that several practitioners carry out an intervention differently. You wonder why this is and when you ask questions in your professional practice, you get different answers!

Example 2: Alternatively, let's imagine you have been asked to write an essay or discuss a case study on a given scenario discussing what you did and why you did it.

For both of the examples above you would need to take an evidence-based approach and ask the question: *'What is the evidence for the way the care was undertaken?'*

To answer this question you would first need to **search for** and **locate** the appropriate evidence. You might find a wide range of different research studies, case studies, guidelines, literature reviews or opinion articles. You would then need to **judge the quality** of the evidence you find and whether it is relevant to your problem or issue. You would probably consider any research that you find to be of more value than someone's personal view. This evidence should then be **applied** to the care of the patient/client, whose needs initiated the question, taking into account their preference and your clinical or professional judgement. The **resources** available may also need to be considered at this point. You may then want to **evaluate** the effectiveness of your intervention in that situation with that patient/client.

We will cover how to ask the right question, how to search for the evidence, and how to judge the value and quality of different types of evidence in more detail later in this book.

This is evidence-based practice in practice!

It is important to find the right evidence to underpin your practice and this book will show you how best to do that. You can see that carrying out an intervention or approach because it has 'always been done' or acting because something is expected of you is not enough. You need to ensure that there are stronger reasons and evidence than acting out of a sense of tradition or ritual. This is not to say that traditional practices are necessarily outdated or to be avoided at all costs. Nor is experience alone to be disregarded. It is just that nowadays, as practitioners, we have a wealth of research available to us which can inform how we should proceed in practice, also considering professional judgement and patient or client preference. Given that we have this opportunity, we need to ensure that we use it for the best outcomes for our patients and clients.

In summary

In this chapter we have discussed the meaning of the term evidence-based practice. We hope that you are now thinking that there is a good logical argument for health and social care to be evidence based. After all, who would want to receive outdated care from a practitioner who could not account for it, in preference to care that is based on the best available evidence combined with professional judgement and patient/client involvement?

In the remainder of this book we will consider why practice needs evidence and what we mean by evidence. We will then consider different research approaches that you might encounter. We will discuss how to search for evidence and then consider how to determine whether it is any good or not. Before that we will consider in more detail why EBP has become so important in our practice today.

Key points

1 There are several reasons why we need to adopt EBP:
   i to ensure best practice
   ii for our professional accountability
   iii to avoid litigation/negligence claims.
2 EBP incorporates using best available evidence, clinical or professional judgement and patient/client preference in our decision making.
3 EBP does not replace using intuition or experience in our practice but can be used alongside them.

2

Where did evidence-based practice come from?

Moving from ritual and traditional approaches • The developing research culture • The on-going information revolution • Why is there so much information available? • So how does this 'information revolution' affect me? • In summary • Key points

In this chapter we will:

- Explore the development of EBP
- Explore the on-going information revolution
- Discuss how this has assisted the transition from reliance on tradition and ritual in our practice towards consideration and use of evidence.

So far we have argued that EBP is an essential approach to the delivery of health and social care. We have discussed how EBP is practice based upon a sound, up-to-date rationale and your own clinical or professional judgement and takes into account the patient/client's wishes. We have also argued that although there are many definitions of EBP and different terms to describe the concept, the central message is consistent throughout:

Use of evidence combined with professional judgement and patient preference should result in high quality care.

We have also discussed how as a student or registered practitioner you need to be able to give reasons for the care you deliver. These ideas probably seem sensible and logical to you as you read this book. However, it is important to acknowledge that EBP is a relatively new concept.

Moving from tradition and ritual towards an evidence-based approach

For many hundreds of years, health and social care practices were based on trial and error, tradition and ritual. Even where an interest in science and research existed, communication was limited so that it was difficult to circulate new ideas and developments, especially on a wide scale.

For many centuries, the concept of *tradition and ritual* dominated health and social care.

Practitioners in the past largely relied on trial and error, following doctor's orders, experience, ritual and what was accepted practice to inform the delivery of care. A culture of research and development had yet to be firmly established within health and social care contexts. You are probably familiar with some popular rituals that were often practised.

Think back to practices that you have previously carried out that are now considered unhelpful or even harmful. If you are a student or new to your profession ask your practice assessor/mentor.

Let's take some **examples** of practices which have been carried out and do not have an evidence base to support them.

Examples from practice:

In many countries, a practice existed whereby female children born to unmarried mothers were removed from their mothers and placed in temporary care. Here convention and social norms of the time were considered more important than the needs of the child and mother. The importance of the mother–child relationship was not considered significant.

> Children in Romania who were failing to thrive were given a small amount of blood in the expectation that this would aid growth. There is no scientific explanation for this and the very sad result is that many children contracted HIV infection from being given infected blood.

From these two examples, you can see that absence of an appropriate evidence base led to practices that we would now consider very harmful.

On a more positive note, the following example illustrates how the development of an evidence-based approach can gradually lead to the reduction of interventions which may be unpleasant or harmful, for which there is not a solid evidence base.

Example from practice:

One example from practice is the idea that children are often advised to have nothing to eat or drink from the midnight before surgery. However, Brady *et al.* (2009) in a review of trials found that drinking clear fluids up to a few hours before surgery did not increase the risk of regurgitation during or after surgery. They noted that there was in fact some benefit preoperatively in terms of thirst and hunger.

Can you identify an area of your own profession, where a change in practice has been recommended due to changes in evidence?

The developing research culture

The research culture within health and social care has become stronger over the past few decades. The concept of 'research-based practice' evolved and practitioners increasingly began to search for a research base for the care they delivered which previously might have been given according to tradition, experience and following orders without question. At the same time, **research education** became a main component of university courses for health and social care professionals at undergraduate and post- graduate levels. Demand for research to underpin practice has increased as more professions moved towards **higher education** rather than on-the-job training or apprenticeship.

For example paramedic services have traditionally worked using an 'on-the-job' training approach. However the recent move to a broader educational focus and courses based in higher education has created a demand for evidence (Petter and Armitage 2012). Whilst some of the practices may not change, it is the shift from anecdotal support of practices to solid reasons that helps develop and keep a professional, safe and effective approach to the role. Also with the development of new evidence, any unsafe, inconsistent and unbeneficial interventions can be avoided.

Over time, the term 'research-based practice' became replaced by 'evidence-based practice' in order to incorporate the influence of professional judgement and patient preference as discussed in Chapter 1. Now we see the influence of EBP on a world-wide scale, as recognition of the value of research and evidence impacts on health systems and public health internationally (Theobald *et al.* 2011; Gilson *et al.* 2011). We have conferences, journals, websites, organizations and institutions all devoted to the concept of EBP.

For example, in January 2011, **The Cochrane Collaboration** (the organization that promotes the publication of high quality systematic reviews) was accepted as a non-governmental organization in **official relations with the World Health Organization** (WHO), the public health arm of the United Nations, establishing formalized communication between both organizations. This partnership promotes collaboration and high-quality research between both organizations to produce evidence to ensure policies in all sectors contribute to improving health and health equity. See http://www.cochrane.org/about-us/relations-world-health-organization for more information.

The result is that we now have a large evidence base upon which to base our practice, although some areas of health and social care are very well researched while others remain under-researched.

Some examples of evidence that have contributed to an evidence-based approach and changes in practice

Example 1: Birnbaum and Saini (2012) recently undertook a review of qualitative studies exploring whether children wanted to be involved in custody decisions post separation or divorce and they found that children generally want to be engaged in the decision-making process regarding custody and access, even if they are not making the final decisions. The suggestion is that social workers provide space for listening to the views of children in this aspect of their work.

Example 2: In a review of quantitative studies, Stead *et al.* (2008) brought together evidence about smoking cessation and summarized that 'advice from doctors helps people who smoke to quit'. Even brief, simple advice about quitting smoking helps people to successfully quit and remain non-smokers 12 months later. This could have massive implications for a cost effective, widely beneficial and quick intervention.

Example 3: The following example comes from the medical treatment of breast cancer but is used here as it illustrates the points we are making. If we look back 50 years, the best known treatment for breast cancer was a full mastectomy, which entailed the total removal of the breast. This was the standard treatment for many years. In the 1970s scientists began to consider whether such radical treatment was indeed the best option and commenced trials to compare whether removal of the malignant lump would be as effective as removal of the whole breast. Many very large studies (known as randomized controlled trials, which we discuss in Chapter 5) were conducted across Europe and within the United States of America and the results of these studies confirmed that in fact it was both safe and effective to remove just the lump rather than the whole breast. As a result of these many studies, practitioners were able to inform patient/clients that a full mastectomy was no longer necessary and the best possible treatment, in most instances became the removal of the lump only. We can therefore see that as a result of these studies, it was possible to establish best practice for the management of breast cancer. The results of these studies led to radical changes in the way that breast cancer was managed.

These are just some examples of research that has led to changes in practice and has contributed to the development of EBP.

The on-going information revolution

The amount of information available to practitioners is now so vast that it can seem impossible to keep on top of. This information is also expanding on a daily basis.

As a health or social care practitioner you may feel overwhelmed by the vast amount of information, of varying quality, which relates to many different specialties and topics. As increasing amounts of research and other information become more readily available, it is increasingly hard to keep abreast of new developments. In fact one group of researchers calculated the number of new journal articles published in a particular area on a weekly basis and came to the conclusion that keeping up to date, let alone being an 'expert' on a topic, had become an impossible expectation (Fraser and Dunstan 2010).

Think about how much easier it must have been before there was so much available evidence upon which to base health and social care.

Maybe there were one or two text books for you to read, rather than the many journals and e-books that are now available to you.

One consequence of the information revolution is that there is also a vast amount of unconfirmed and unreliable information around. There is a lot of information that is misleading or based on unhelpful assumptions, such as myths, rumours and 'word on the street'. It is vital that as a practitioner you do not perpetuate these ideas. We discuss how you identify good quality evidence from poorer quality evidence in Chapter 6. As a health and social care practitioner you have to consider all the information and evidence you come across and work out which is useful to you. Goldacre (2008) illustrates many examples of a non-evidence-based approach in his book entitled *Bad Science*. In this book and on his web site (http://www.badscience.net/), he explores and often exposes health and social care stories which are presented or reported as fact that are based on very little, inaccurate or no evidence. For example in his book he dedicates a chapter to homeopathy and, more recently, on his website discusses claims made regarding the role of vitamin supplements in the treatment of HIV and AIDs, and claims that traditional treatments for these diseases were harmful.

Goldacre illustrates clearly that the vast amount of information available needs close scrutiny. There is also some concern that practitioners might be tempted to ignore the growing evidence base and continue to use outdated practices. Ernst (2008) summarizes some concerning events in which institutions disregarded evidence when it didn't suit their policy or commercial interests. We have outlined the likely consequences of this in Chapter 1. It is clearly within your role as a health and social care practitioner to get behind the headlines and simple reports so that you are not supporting claims that do not have a sound evidence base.

Why is there so much information available?

There are two main reasons why there is so much available evidence:

- **Increased demand for research and more/better quality research being produced.**
- **Information is more widely available from the Internet.**

Increased demand for research and more and better quality research is being produced

We have discussed the increased demand for research and the development of the concept of EBP which has arisen as health and social care practitioners move away from a traditional approach to care delivery, towards an evidence-based approach. This has led to an enormous number of publications and the development of research organizations such as the **Cochrane Collaboration** and **Campbell Collaboration** as mentioned in Chapter 1. You only have to look at the titles of journals in any library collection to see the range of journals that relate to a particular professional field. In addition, some of these journals may be published on a weekly or monthly basis. It can seem an impossible task to keep up to date with new developments, even within your own area, without developing strategies for managing the information which we will discuss later in this chapter.

However this is not to say that you will always find evidence to underpin your practice. There are important areas that have not been researched. All research needs to be approved by appropriate ethical bodies prior to commencement and it can take years after the successful award of a research grant before the research is undertaken. This is because research is a complex and lengthy process that can take some time to get started.

Example from practice:

You might be surprised to read that, at the time of writing, for example, despite the widespread concern about a 'flu pandemic and the availability of the anti-viral drug 'Tamiflu', there is no evidence from large-scale studies about the actual effectiveness of the drug (Yong 2012). Writing in the *British Medical Journal*, Yong describes the need to **'fast track'** certain **research projects** to ensure that evidence is available at the time that it is required.

Information is more widely available from the Internet, mobile devices and social media

The second reason for this increase in available information is the dramatic increase in **information technology** which has led to the increasing availability of information. Before the advent of this technology, libraries contained hard-bound indexes and volumes of the journals that were likely to be most relevant to their students. Practitioners would probably subscribe locally to relevant professional journals and even have their own departmental libraries. This restricted the breadth of what was available. Consequently, there were always a large number of journals that were not available to staff and students or available only through inter-library loan. This meant that it was difficult and expensive to access relevant information.

With the advent of online libraries, databases and journals, students and practitioners have access to many thousands of journals and e-books in addition to websites and other sources of information and references. The way people communicate and access information is changing rapidly from a planned, static approach to the expectation that information can be accessed spontaneously, anywhere and immediately. Whilst this is advantageous to health and social care practitioners (notwithstanding the problem of information overload), it is also of benefit to patients as social media and information technology has been used for the benefit of patient information systems.

Examples from practice:

Example 1: Fisher and Clayton (2012) carried out a small local survey in the USA and concluded that there is growing patient acceptance of social media in healthcare. They concluded that professionals should gain understanding of the type of people using it, their preferences, and the barriers to using it so that providers can prioritize effort when using evidence-based social media in their practice.

Example 2: Text messaging has also been used especially with children and adolescents (Militello *et al.* 2012). It has been found that mobile phones are ideal in reaching all demographics and that interventions using short messages may be most effective as a reminder to support disease management behaviours. Research in this area and information communicated by a variety of social media formats is likely to increase.

So how does this 'information revolution' affect me?

In short, as practitioners we have a duty to incorporate evidence-based information into our everyday practice to enhance patient/client care. As we have already discussed, practitioners are accountable for their practice and this requirement has grown with the increasing amount of information that is available regarding health and social care. In addition to the information available to professionals, our patients/clients are more able to access information too and so may want to be involved more in decision making. As the available information increases, it is more and more likely that there will be some good quality research available that underpins the care or treatment you deliver. Therefore if you practise as you have always done in the past without seeking to update yourself, it is likely that you will find that your practice is out of date and there is evidence to support a different way of doing things. You may then be called to account as to why your practice is out of date, or, if you give advice or an intervention that is not based on evidence you are more likely to be challenged by fellow practitioners or patients/clients. With the on-going information revolution, keeping up to date with new ideas and research is arguably more difficult than it was previously.

How can I manage the increasing information that I will come across?

It is easy to feel overwhelmed by the amount of evidence available on a topic. Smith (2010) discusses some possible responses to this information overload, including a 'head in the sand strategy' and reliance on information gained from other colleagues. There are ways to manage the information overload, such as using systematic reviews, good quality literature reviews and research-based guidelines and policy. We will discuss other strategies that you might use to keep up to date with the ever-increasing amount of evidence available in Chapter 7.

In summary

The on-going information revolution presents a challenge to all who practise within health and social care. No longer is it acceptable to say *'this is how I've always done this'* and to carry on with an out-dated practice in the light of new evidence. The increase in the amount of available evidence and the ways that this can be accessed, together with the demand and drive for research evidence, have led to an expectation and culture in which practice is founded on evidence. You will as a student or qualified practitioner need to be able to justify the care that you give. In the remainder of this book, we will explore how you can best access, evaluate and make sense of the information that is available to you. In Chapter 5, we discuss how to search for relevant information and evidence. In Chapter 6 we discuss how you can identify whether or not the evidence you find is useful. Finally in Chapter 7 we discuss strategies for adopting an evidence-based approach, and what the realities of that are like, within the realistic context of busy professional practice.

Key points

1 It is no longer acceptable to base our practice on tradition or ritual.
2 The dramatic rise in the quantity, quality and availability of information has led to the need to incorporate this information into daily practice.
3 Use of good quality, up-to-date evidence is expected by our patients/clients and we are accountable for ensuring we use it.

3

Using evidence in your decision making and to answer practical questions

Evidence and decision making • The consequences and implications of your decision • What types of evidence do we need to make different decisions? • What kind of evidence is available? • Finding the right type of research evidence • Research that is directly applicable • Research that has not been conducted in your setting • What other 'evidence' is there out there? • In summary • Key points

In this chapter we will consider:

- When do we need to use evidence?
- What types of evidence are available to help us make decisions?
- What do we do when there is limited evidence?

We will consider how to search for evidence in detail in Chapter 5. We will discuss in greater detail how you make sense of and apply the evidence you find in Chapters 6 and 7.

If, before you started reading this book, you thought that EBP was something that concerned only the highest level decisions in health and social care, you will now be fully aware that it is something that affects all practitioners, at all levels of service provision.

In simple terms, every time you undertake a professional activity or decision, you need to ask yourself what evidence you need to act in that situation.

Evidence and decision making

We make decisions all the time in all professional areas. Let's look at the decision-making process so we can see where the components of evidence based practice fit in. Hastie and Dawes (2010) state that decision making is made up of three parts:

- There has to be more than once course of action.
- The decision maker considers the possible or expected outcomes.
- The consequences are assessed of each possible outcome based on personal beliefs and goals.

Recognizing that there is more than one possible course of action is part of making a professional judgement. Evidence is then used to consider the expected outcomes of the decision and the possible consequences.

Standing (2005: 34 and 2010) has defined decision making as:

A complex process involving information processing, critical thinking, evaluating evidence, applying relevant knowledge, problem solving skills, reflection and clinical judgement to select the best course of action which optimises a patient/client's health and minimises any potential harm . . .

You can see how both definitions of decision making incorporate the need for EBP – that is, using the best available evidence, together with professional judgement and taking consideration of patient/client preference. So the link between EBP and decision making is clear.

There are many different activities and decisions that require the use of evidence. Thompson and Stapley (2011) highlighted several decision types:

- Decisions about interventions
- Decisions about which patients or clients will benefit most from an intervention
- Decisions about the best time to intervene
- Decisions about when to deliver information
- Decisions about how to manage a service or care delivery
- Decisions about how to reassure patients and clients.

In the reality of practice there may be overlap and decision types may not be so clear cut as you will see from our examples below. We have described some of the varied decisions you may have to make and the different types of evidence you may draw upon in the examples below:

Examples of different decisions

Example: If you are a midwife, you might regularly give advice about breast feeding. Some mothers might be struggling to breast feed and you might be tempted to suggest supplementing with bottle feeding as you have heard others do. You need to check the evidence behind this and ensure that you give the best available advice to new mothers and their babies. In this case, the evidence you need is research that addresses the best form of nutrition for new born babies.

Example: If you are a social worker, you might regularly need to assess risk of depression in clients and you need to be able to suggest effective strategies to support your client. In this case, the evidence you need is research that addresses the types of interventions that are effective.

Example: If you are a surgical nurse, you might regularly need to give an intramuscular injection and you need to know the best site for the injection and the best technique to use. In this case, the evidence you need is evidence which addresses the most appropriate site for giving an injection.

Example: If you are an occupational therapist, you might regularly need to discuss fall prevention strategies with clients. In this case, the evidence you need is that which is concerned with effectiveness of different fall prevention strategies.

Example: If you are a physiotherapist, you might regularly give advice to clients with tendonitis and need to know about the effects of exercise versus rest versus alternative strategies. In this case, the evidence you need is that which has evaluated the effectiveness of various interventions for tendonitis.

Example: If you are working with vulnerable people, you might regularly need to monitor the fluid intake of your clients to ensure they do not suffer from dehydration. You notice that one client is not drinking a lot of fluid. In this case, the evidence you need is about the importance of adequate hydration.

The consequences and implications of your decision

Some decisions will be more important than others. This will depend on the nature of the **risk** or ***potential for harm*** involved to the patient/client in undertaking or omitting the intervention and the cost involved.

In the examples given above, we have identified examples where the decisions to be made have serious implications. If mothers and babies are not appropriately supported in breast feeding, the longer term health of the baby may suffer. If the occupational therapist does not give appropriate advice regarding falls prevention, a patient or client may have a serious accident. Even if the decision does not appear life threatening – for example, the management of tendonitis – these conditions can have serious impact on the quality of the person's life.

Consider the areas in your own professional practice. Can you identify higher risk activities? Are these activities or interventions based on evidence?

Below, we have given an example of a decision which most people would probably consider to have few implications and an example of a decision which most people would probably consider to be more serious.

Example 1: A person with high blood pressure asks you if there is any truth in the idea that eating garlic can reduce blood pressure. This is a low risk intervention – people eat garlic all the time and there are no known disadvantages in doing so. As a low risk intervention, investigation would probably not ordinarily be your priority. However the patient's confidence in you is likely to be improved if you refer to recent evidence. In a systematic review, Stabler *et al.* (2012) found that, although there may be some benefit for some patients, there is currently not enough high quality information so the patient could make a decision to try it and see if it worked for them.

Example 2: A person in a health or social care setting notices that not all staff are washing their hands between each patient or client that they look after. The decision of the healthcare provider to omit hand hygiene is a high risk omission. There is evidence that all health and social care practitioners should thoroughly decontaminate their hands between every episode of patient/client contact. The evidence is very strong that hand cleansing is probably the most important strategy in infection control and this has been shown in many large reviews of research studies, for example Jefferson *et al.* (2011). This is an inexpensive task but a highly effective one which can have serious consequences if not meticulously followed. Thus, failure to follow this EBP would be very difficult, if not impossible, to justify.

Identifying importance and urgency in decision making

We have illustrated that some decisions might be more significant than others and that the decision to respond to a patient or client's request for information about the use of garlic in the prevention of high blood pressure might be less important or urgent than other decisions you might make. However it is very difficult to assess the urgency or importance of decisions we make – what is important to one person may be less important to another and so on. If we are to adopt an EBP approach then clearly, if there is good available evidence about the decision you need to make, then you should use this in your decision making if your professional judgement, circumstances, patient preference and resources permit. The greater the risk to the patient/client or likelihood of harm, the more important it is that our practice is based on evidence. However it is good practice to consider the evidence base behind all of the practice we undertake.

Finding out that there is *no available research evidence,* rather than assuming that there is none, is very valuable information which you can use to justify why you need to use other forms of evidence.

What types of evidence do we need to make different decisions?

Just as there are many types of decisions that you make on a daily basis, there are also many types of evidence you will use to underpin those decisions.

In general terms, you should adopt the most appropriate care and be able to justify it with reference to *the most appropriate* evidence.

Evidence will often be from **primary research** or better still **reviews of research.** This is because research provides direct observation of the effect of interventions and care procedures on the patient/clients and clients themselves or as in the case of qualitative research, provides us with insight so that we may more fully understand a situation or the service users' experiences. Ideally, this research will form the basis of **policy and guidelines** or **care pathways.** You might also draw on **local policy,** which has been developed for the management of complex situations. If there is no research evidence, you might draw on established scientific information and use this evidence to make reasoned deductions about what you need to know. In addition, we can draw on sociology and psychology to help us make decisions. The evidence you will be looking for will be from a varied range of sources. Sometimes you will not look to research to make your decision but would need different evidence, for example policy documents, legal precedents, or ethical principles. Whether or not we define policy, law and ethics as 'evidence' is something that could be debated. However they certainly amount to rationale from which we draw to inform our practice. Your practice would not withstand scrutiny if you relied on out-dated policy, or unlawful or unethical practice.

Professional practice in all areas can be very complex. Standing (2008) argues that there are likely to be many other factors that you consider when making a decision and it will depend on the complexity of the decision and the time available. Standing has developed a continuum that illustrates how if you have sufficient time available to you and the appropriate resources, you will be able to make a considered and rational decision, fully informed by relevant evidence. If you have less time and there is a moment of crisis, your decision is likely to be more reactionary. This is where the use of policy and guidelines are useful as they provide guidance in a situation where you need to make a quick decision. You are also likely to draw on **patient/client opinion**, your own intuition and **reflective judgement**, and the **expertise of others** when you make a complex decision in a specific context – particularly where there are time pressures. These constitute the **clinical or professional judgement** component of EBP.

Standing (2010) argues that the role of the decision maker is to be professionally accountable for assessing patient/clients' needs using **appropriate sources of information** and planning interventions that address their problems. In the examples we give throughout this chapter we will emphasize that there are many different types of evidence that you will draw on in your professional decision making.

Let's have a look at some of the decisions you are likely to be faced with in everyday practice. You will see that the type of evidence needed to make the decisions come from a range of sources, not just research evidence.

Examples of decisions and the type of evidence they require

Decision 1: My patient/client has been diagnosed as an alcoholic and wants to self-discharge against the judgement of staff. What should I do?

*Evidence you need to help you make a decision – you would need relevant **legal and ethical principles** regarding the right of the patient/client to discharge and the duty owed to him by the health or social care practitioner. Local **policy** may also guide this decision. You may also use **professional judgement** and **prior experience** in exploring with him the options for his care. You might refer to your **professional body standards** too.*

Decision 2: A mature student on placement has considerable personal issues and they don't appear to be coping well. How shall I handle it?

Evidence you need to help you make decision – *you would need to find out the university policy on supporting students, you may seek the views of your colleagues or the expert opinion of a tutor. You may also use your intuition and experience to help you respond to particular issues. You could find qualitative research that explores the mature student experience of placements.*

Decision 3: My patient/client has asked me about the use of acupuncture as a pain-relieving agent. What should I advise?

Evidence you need to help you make a decision – *to answer any questions about the effectiveness of an intervention, you would need to find research, ideally in the form of systematic reviews or randomized controlled trials that have looked specifically at the issue in question (we will discuss what randomized controlled trials are and why they are needed later on).*

Decision 4: A client with depression wants to have greater access to his children. How can I best support him?

Evidence you need to help you make a decision – *you would need to explore the client's rights as a father from a legal perspective, and the implications of his depression on his ability to care for his children which may come from qualitative research about the experiences of those with depression coping with parenthood.*

Decision 5: I want to know if I should expel the air bubble in a syringe of Fragmin (a drug to reduce the incidence of deep vein thrombosis) before administering an injection. What should I do?

Evidence you need to help you make a decision – *you would search to see if there is any research evidence, but in the absence of this you should examine up-to-date manufacturers' instructions on their website http://www.fragmin. com/assets/pdfs/Fragmin_ClinicDosing&AdminBroch.pdf and look to see if there is any rationale given. In this case the air bubble ensures the full dose of the drug is given.*

Decision 6: My patient/client with cognitive impairment seems restless and I am wondering if I should ensure they are given their 'as required' pain medication?

Evidence you need to help you make a decision – *you could search the literature on 'pain assessment in cognitively impaired adults'. You may find validated assessment tools or advice on how best to assess this client group. You could discuss the behaviour with family/carers to see if it is indicative of pain. You could use other physiological measurements such as pulse and blood pressure recordings to assess the individual. You may find studies that report that pain is generally underassessed and treated in those with cognitive impairment.*

You can see from the examples that we make decisions in a wide variety of contexts and that a variety of forms of evidence are needed. When you are looking for evidence on your topic, 'one size' really does not fit all. If anyone tells you that you *always need research evidence* to answer your question, this would be misleading – you need the most relevant information that will answer your question. This is often research but as we have seen in the previous examples, it might come from another source, for example policy, or legal or ethical principles. In a busy professional context, when you are managing complex situations, you may find that there is no easy fit between the evidence and the environment you are working in. The type of evidence you need depends on the decision you have to make and you need to think carefully about this to work out the type of evidence you need.

When you seek out evidence to use in your practice, it is sometimes referred to as practising in an 'evidence informed way'. The difficulty is that no one can tell you what type of evidence you need in a given situation; you need to use your own judgement to work this out.

Getting started: defining your question or decision

You should start by clarifying and narrowing down the question or exact decision you need to make. In order to do this, the first thing you need to do is **define a question/refine the decision** that identifies what you need to know. This is important because unless you are focussed, you will not be able to work out how to find the information and you will be swamped with information. You are therefore likely to end up more confused than when you started! We will discuss this in more detail in Chapter 5.

Example: A friend asks about anti-malarial tablets as she is about to go off on a foreign adventure. Where would you start?

First of all, you would need to clarify exactly what your friend wants to know. What question are they asking of you? Are they concerned about . . .

- The effectiveness of the various types of anti-malarial tablets on the market?
- The health and environmental effects of the tablets?
- The cost?
- The best time to travel to avoid mosquitoes?
- People's experiences of using the various tablets?

If you do not identify exactly what your friend wants to know you will not be able to find the appropriate evidence to advise them in a meaningful way. You might find out which is the most effective whilst what they really wanted to know was which is the cheapest. The information you do find is likely to be of limited usefulness if it doesn't find out what your friend wanted to know.

The message is clear – you need to know what the question is before you begin to look for the right type of evidence.

If you are looking for evidence about the effectiveness of anti-malarial tablets, this evidence will not be the same as that you would look for if you were looking for evidence about the experiences of those who have used the different tablets.

What kind of evidence is available?

There are many decisions and many different kinds of evidence that will assist your decision making. As we have said before, evidence comes in many forms. What would be weak evidence for one decision would be stronger evidence for another decision. Think back to the six decisions, described earlier, that needed evidence. Different types of evidence were needed to assist with decision making – legal rulings, policy and guidelines and research evidence.

Anecdotal evidence

You are probably familiar with the term anecdotal evidence. This is generally a weaker form of evidence for all types of decisions for the reasons outlined below. However if no other evidence is available you might consider that anecdotal evidence is the best available evidence to use.

Example: Imagine you are trying to train your dog. He is not an easy dog to train – he is somewhat feisty and pulls on the lead. You try out a few choker collars which pull tighter around his neck when he pulls and relaxes when he walks nicely to heel. You aim to see which one he responds to the best. You find one that seems to be a good fit and deters him from pulling on the lead. Here you have some evidence about which choker lead works best – at least for you and your dog. This is anecdotal evidence and is the type of evidence that people have gathered and used over the generations. Indeed a lot of health and social care has been based on anecdotal evidence in the absence of harder evidence being available. Now imagine that you have hundreds of dogs at a Guide Dog training centre and you need to know which lead works the best. **Here the stakes are higher for many reasons:**

- The effective training of the dogs is even more important because of the role they are to perform.
- The cost of the lead must be multiplied by the number of dogs so there is a big cost implication.
- The time taken to train the dog also has cost implications.

If you were a recipient of a guide dog or a donator to the charitable organization Guide Dogs for the Blind, you would want to know that the best lead was being used to train the dogs. In this instance, the anecdotal evidence gained from the experience of one person attempting to train his dog would not seem sufficient. You would want more robust evidence upon which to base your choice of dog lead.

This scenario can be transferred to health and social care settings in which the stakes are high. There are limited resources and patients/clients have an expectation and a right to receive the optimum care. We cannot afford to get it wrong. Anecdotal evidence – or trial and error – is clearly not enough. We cannot afford to base practice on insubstantial evidence which does not stand up to scrutiny.

In health and social care, **anecdotal evidence** can be:

- Using something you've tried before that worked and you haven't checked out whether there is an evidence base to support this.
- From your colleague or practice assessor/mentor who says 'we've always done it like this'
- From discussion papers, opinion articles or editorials
- Expert opinion (consultants, specialist practitioners, other colleagues, although their opinion is very likely to be informed by evidence – but do not make this assumption!).

In principle, you should be aware that the quality of evidence provided by anecdotal information – even if it is based on expert opinion – is generally weaker than that which is provided by research or reviews of research. Remember that if you do not ask for the evidence that lies behind the advice you are given, you might be practising using anecdotal evidence only and your practice would not stand up to scrutiny. However, published material that does not report research findings can still be useful. This is why it is important to determine what evidence you need in the first instance. Anecdotal information can be useful in the following ways:

- It can contribute to your professional judgement.
- It can be used to set the context/give background information.
- It can be used to identify what common practice is in the light of little other evidence.
- It might be used to give insight to your research question directly if there is minimal research on the topic.
- It might also be used directly to address the research question, for example, if you are specifically looking at how the media portrays the role of the occupational therapist, then media cuttings will be of utmost relevance to your review.

In the same way that the Guide Dog trainer needs good evidence about the effectiveness of the different dog leads available, so the health and social care provider needs good evidence about the effectiveness of the care they deliver. With the availability of systematic and rigorous research studies, we now have more robust evidence upon which to base our practice.

Finding the right type of research evidence for your decision or question

So if we need to move away from anecdotal evidence, what do we move towards?

It is important that we use the *right evidence for the question we want to answer.*

In Chapter 4, we discuss the different types of research in detail. For the flow of argument in this book, we want to discuss some more general principles and ideas about research before we go into detail about the specific studies themselves. However if any of the following examples do not make complete sense without additional information, do refer to Chapter 4. In the following examples, we refer to some of the types of research in order to illustrate the point that different research is needed to answer different questions and that 'one size does not fit all'.

Evidence about 'does it work or not?'

If you need to know about the effectiveness of an intervention or therapy, the only way to really tell if something is effective is to find a study (or review of studies) that has directly compared one thing to another. We call this type of study a 'randomized controlled trial' (RCT). This is because in an RCT there is an intervention group and a control group who do not receive the intervention in question who act as a direct comparison. Unless you have a direct comparison, you cannot really tell if something works or not. Therefore in this case, RCTs are the 'gold standard' of evidence you are looking for. However don't let anyone tell you that RCTs are the 'gold standard' of evidence for every information need. RCTs only help you if you are looking at whether a treatment or care method is effective. If you are not looking at effectiveness, then RCTs will not be the 'gold standard' evidence for your question. If your friend in the example above wants to know which anti-malarial tablets are the most effective, you would need to look for an RCT which had compared one tablet against another.

If the manufacturers are telling you that their product is effective, but you cannot find an independent RCT to back this up, then you should be wary of that claim!

Evidence about 'what is it like?'

If you are looking for evidence about people's experience – such as users' experience of insect repellents, an RCT is unlikely to help you, unless you found one that compared the users' experience of one type against another. Instead, you could look for research reports that explore the person's experience, or a review of such research. This is likely to be through asking them about it using a qualitative approach and probably in-depth interviews. If your friend in the example above wants to know about how other people have experienced a particular anti-malarial tablet and the side-effects, you need to look for research that explores patients' experiences of taking malaria tablets.

Evidence about 'what do they do in practice?'

If you are looking to find out what actually happens in practice – for example, whether people actually take the anti-malarial tablet when they are in a high risk area – you would need to look for studies that directly report use of the prophylaxis. In this situation, this could be difficult to find out exactly how many people adhere to a prophylaxis regime, without undercover observers, which would clearly be impossible! Instead, those concerned with the adherence with the prophylaxis against malaria would need to rely on the patient's own reported adherence to the anti-malarial drugs prescribed. This information might be collected in a survey or interview.

However there are times that you can observe what actually happens in practice.

Example: Imagine that you are concerned about infection in your unit and want to find out about how compliant staff are with hand-washing/hand-rubbing policies. Consider the type of evidence you would you look for. Imagine that you then found a questionnaire study that had asked staff at the end of every shift whether they always follow infection control procedures. Consider the answers they are likely to give and whether these would reflect what they *actually* do. How strong would that evidence be? What type of evidence would you be looking for that would really tell you about staff adherence to infection control policy?

Clearly the answer is to find observational studies, in which an observer has sat and watched to see if staff washed their hands or not in the everyday context. Any evidence that falls short of this approach would not be very strong. Thus for this question, the very best type of evidence would be observational studies. Our recall or description of what we do can be different from what we actually do!

Think about how you could pick an issue in your professional practice and focus your question differently to find different types of evidence.

You can see from these examples that it is helpful to be able to 'pin point' the type of research you are looking for and that different types of research inform us about different aspects of professional practice and decisions that need to be made. We have argued that research evidence is usually the basis of evidence we use in our professional practice. When we are thinking about evidence-based practice, we need to ensure that we use the strongest possible evidence to support our practice. If we do not seek out strong evidence, we risk being criticized for not using up-to-date, robust evidence. Remember that the nature of evidence in health and social care changes very quickly and what was considered good evidence at one time can become quickly outdated. However you must also remember that nothing is perfect and you may not always be able to find strong evidence. You should aim to base your practice on the **best available evidence** you can find.

We will now consider how closely research should be related to your professional environment for it to be useful to you. Ideally you will find research that is directly applicable to your area of professional practice but this will not always be the case.

Research that is directly applicable or highly relevant

Research that is *directly applicable* refers to research evidence that relates directly to the health and social care practice situation you are involved with.

In an ideal world, there would be direct evidence to underpin the care you deliver and this evidence would be based on direct observations or studies of people who are similar to those you look after. Also in an ideal world, you would find that the evidence that exists relates directly to your clinical or professional setting so that you can be as sure as possible that it applies to your patient or client.

An **example** would be that of hand cleansing. The process of hand cleansing is the same whichever patients/clients you work with, except of course that some patients/clients are under additional infection control precautions or the procedures or interventions may be higher or lower risk. Research evidence relating to hand cleansing will be relevant to your practice irrespective of where and when it was undertaken, although of course, you still need to assess the quality of the research undertaken.

A further **example** of direct evidence would be the impact of shift work on the quality of care. Shift work is an integral component of all practice areas where patients/clients require 24-hour care. Thus any research which explores quality of care provision and its relationship to shift work is likely to be directly relevant to all disciplines.

However, more often than not, you will come across evidence that does not relate directly to your patient/client or client group or the exact situation you encounter. This evidence can still be useful to you as discussed below.

Research that has not been conducted in your particular setting or with your patient or client group

There will be much research available that has not been conducted specifically with your patient or client group or in your professional setting but is nonetheless relevant to you. The research might have been carried out on a different group of patients or clients or in a different country, so its relevance and application to your setting might be different.

For example, this research could include:

• Research undertaken with patient or client groups in a related area
• Research that has been undertaken in a laboratory
• Research from other academic disciplines

Research undertaken with patients or clients groups in a related area

For example, consider some research about how information giving reduces anxiety. Let's say that you come across some research that was undertaken with patients/clients in an oncology ward. You are working in general surgery. This evidence will be less directly relevant to your patients/clients and you need to determine the extent to which the research is relevant to you. We will discuss ways of assessing the quality of the evidence further on in this book but for now it is important to note that you are likely to have to make a judgement about the applicability of the evidence you encounter to your professional practice. This is the 'clinical/professional judgement' component of EBP we referred to in Chapter 1. However this research may be relevant to you in some way. This is why we refer to it as indirect evidence.

Alternatively, imagine you are working with deprived children in an inner city from a particular cultural group. There is research evidence about the most effective way to promote uptake of day care provision that has been undertaken with a different cultural group but nothing that relates to the particular group of children you are working with. Again, this is where your clinical or professional judgement comes into play. You might find that this is the best available evidence and you need to determine how relevant it is to the group of children you are working with.

You are probably thinking by now that much of the evidence you use in your practice is indirect evidence – that is, even if it was obtained through direct observation or experiments on patient or clients, its focus was not on the practice setting you are working in and therefore the evidence does not apply to your practice directly and you have to make a judgement about its relevance to your practice area. You will find that this is often the case.

Consider why research that was carried out in the USA on the funding of health and social care might not be relevant, yet research carried out on a therapeutic activity may be relevant.

This may be because the health and social care funding systems are very different in the USA, but the effectiveness of an intervention may be just as effective on people with similar issues or problems in both countries. You need to judge if it is relevant or not.

Research undertaken in a laboratory

It might be that you find that there is no research that is directly applicable or that which you can apply to your own professional context. It will often be the case that there is insufficient direct or indirectly applicable research evidence available to you about the specific question you are investigating. This does not mean that you cannot practise EBP. You can still find evidence to underpin your practice, even if it is not immediately obvious what information might be relevant to you. Sometimes, the results of research undertaken in a laboratory might be relevant to our professional practice. For example, consider the use of antiseptic skin wash prior to surgery. There is no strong evidence to suggest that use of a skin wash prior to surgery reduces post-operative infection. However there is evidence from the laboratory that use of antiseptic solutions used on the skin do lower the bacterial count – as you might expect. Therefore the practice of asking patients to wash with an antiseptic prior to surgery is based on laboratory research, rather than direct research undertaken in practice.

Evidence deduced from research undertaken in laboratory conditions can be applied to professional practice.

Your practice can be underpinned by evidence which is deduced from scientific knowledge rather than from research studies that have been carried out on patients/clients directly

It is often necessary to look further afield for sources that might provide you with an evidence base for your practice. This is because professional practice encompasses a very wide range of activities and will therefore draw on a wide range of sources of evidence to justify practice. Evidence deduced from scientific knowledge is evidence which is obtained from scientific and social scientific explanations about how things work, but which have not been tested or observed scientifically (empirically) with patient or clients in the practice setting. By scientific knowledge we mean from the hard sciences, such as biology, physiology and also from social sciences such as sociology and psychology.

Research adopted from other disciplines

At other times we can use research evidence from other disciplines to provide rationale for our practice. Take for example, the practice of taking the patient's or client's physiological observations. We know from our understanding of physiology that taking the patient/client's vital signs – temperature, pulse and blood pressure – will give an indication of the condition of the patient/client. We also know that low blood pressure readings are indicative of haemorrhage. There is, therefore, a physiological rationale for taking a patient/client's blood pressure following surgery. Yet in order to really know how effective this practice is in the prevention and management of haemorrhage we would need to observe the effectiveness of this in practice. Recently there have been concerns that although staff take observations, they are not acting quickly enough on abnormal results and so many institutions have set up guidelines and checklists such as early warning scoring systems as advised by the NICE pathway (2012) (available at http://pathways.nice.org.uk/pathways/acutely-ill-patients-in-hospital).

Another example of knowledge which is drawn from a wider body of evidence is the practice of laying out a patient shortly after death. If we look at the wider psychological and sociological literature surrounding dignity, grief and coping with the loss of a loved one, we would find evidence for the practice.

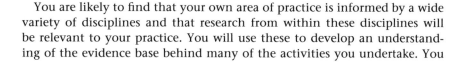

All our professions rely on knowledge from many different disciplines, including sociology and psychology and pharmacology to name but a few.

You are likely to find that your own area of practice is informed by a wide variety of disciplines and that research from within these disciplines will be relevant to your practice. You will use these to develop an understanding of the evidence base behind many of the activities you undertake. You might therefore need to think quite broadly to find evidence to justify your practice.

 What other specialist disciplines predominantly inform your professional practices?

If you do this you may be able to identify the direct and indirect sources of research evidence that influence your practice.

> **Sciences from which we might draw evidence might include:**
>
> Physiology and patho-physiology, medicine (many branches), pharmacology, sociology, immunology, dietetics, radiology, epidemiology, cytology, microbiology, gerontology, anatomy, psychiatry, psychology, podiatry.

What other 'evidence' is there out there?

You will not always find direct or indirect research information on your topic – either a literature review or individual pieces of research. Imagine a line where traditional practices and ritual were at one end and a fully evidence-based approach was at the other.

ritualistic practice   evidence-based practice

◄───►

You would probably like to think that the majority of health and social care interventions fall at the evidence-based end of the continuum. However, unfortunately there are still some areas where there is a lack of research and as can be seen from a high number of Cochrane and Campbell reviews, in some cases the quality of research is not good enough to draw conclusions from and so more or higher quality research is needed.

No research evidence at all?

As we discussed in Chapter 2, sometimes you may not find any research-based information, or you might not be in a position to identify the best possible evidence. As we suggested earlier in this chapter, in this case you will rely on other sources of knowledge and evidence, such as experience, advice from colleagues (think back to the 'Cognitive Continuum' referred to earlier in this chapter) that describes reflective judgement, patient and peer-aided judgement and intuition. You should be aware that depending on the task, time issue or problem these sources may provide a weaker source of evidence.

You should always try to avoid relying on sources of information where the author, the credibility of the information or date of publication is unclear, such as those you might come across on the internet.

If you think about your own everyday practice, how much do you think should or can be based on actual high quality evidence?

The best evidence to look for:

- **Systematic literature reviews** – probably the most important single source of evidence, we will explain why in the next chapter.
- **Research papers** – remember that all topics are diverse and you need to find a paper that looks at your particular research interest – that is, a research paper that explores whether a new intervention is acceptable to patients or clients is very different from one that explores whether it works! Make sure the aim of the research paper reflects your own information needs.

Evidence to be cautious of:

- **Evidence obtained through broad use of search engines.** Beware of sources retrieved through random **search engine** searches such as **Google.**
- **Unknown websites.** Websites can be useful. We will discuss this in Chapter 6. However, it is vital that you assess the sources upon which the website is based.
- **Wikipedia.** The information on Wikipedia is placed there by the public. Whilst it can be useful to provide explanations and sometimes useful key authors names, it should not be relied upon. It may help you identify key search terms to use on more reliable databases.
- **One single piece of non-research based evidence that makes a claim about practice.** This might be an opinion piece found in a professional journal. We will consider how to judge the quality of the evidence that you find in Chapter 6 but the point we would like to make here is that one piece of literature, even research, is rarely enough for you to base your practice on.
- **What your colleagues, practice assessors/mentors say.** Although much learning occurs from the sharing of information from those who are more experienced to those with less experience or skill, you should adopt a critical approach in accepting this information as evidence – especially when the source of knowledge cannot be stated.

In summary

Every time you make a decision you need to consider the evidence base you can draw on to make the decision. Asking your colleague or practice assessor/

mentor is not enough! Research-based evidence should normally be drawn on in the first instance and this may be linked directly or less directly to your area of practice. If no research evidence is available, then you will draw on weaker evidence. It is important to recognize how strong the evidence is that you draw upon as this reflects how much confidence you can have in the evidence you use.

Key points

1 Every time you make a decision, you need to consider what evidence you need to base your decision upon.
2 There are many different types of decision and many different types of evidence to use.
3 You will **normally** use research evidence in the first instance.
4 At other times you will need a different rationale – for example ethical principles or legal guidance.
5 Some research will be directly relevant to your question; other research will be less directly relevant.
6 You might also use physiological, psychological, sociological, pharmaco-logical evidence or where relevant theory, reflective judgement or intuition.
7 Policy and guidelines should be based on research evidence.
8 Use anecdotal evidence as a last resort.

4

What are the different types of research and how do they help us answer different questions?

*How do I recognize research? • Systematic reviews and good quality
literature reviews • Quantitative research • Experimental and non-
experimental quantitative research • Qualitative studies • Different
approaches to qualitative research • Which type of research is best? •
What does the term 'hierarchy of evidence' mean? • What about using
secondary sources? • Use of policy and guidelines • Non-research based
evidence • In summary • Key points*

In the previous chapter, we provided a broad overview of the different kinds
of evidence that are available to assist you when using an evidence-based
approach to your practice. In this chapter we will consider:

- The different types of research in detail and other evidence that you might
  find
- How the question you want to answer influences the type of evidence you
  look for

acknowledge that EBP does not necessarily mean that you will always be using research evidence – but this is often the case. Therefore, given that research can be hard to understand, we have devoted this chapter to summarizing what types of research evidence you are likely to encounter. We advise that you dip in and out of this chapter regarding specific research methods when you need to find out about them.

How do I recognize research?

Research is generally recognizable by the way it is presented. Research normally begins with a question, then a description of how the study was conducted followed by the results and conclusion. The research methods outlined below are just some of the methods that you might encounter. It is important that you are familiar with the different approaches to research design so that you can judge the relevance and quality of it. We will discuss this in greater detail in Chapter 6.

Brainstorm the research methods that you have heard of.

The **research evidence** you might come across can be classified as follows:

- **Systematic reviews or good quality literature reviews**
- **Quantitative research** (sometimes called **primary research**), of which there are many different types but classified into:
  - **Experimental methods** (where an intervention is given to one group and not to another and the outcomes observed), for example, randomized controlled trials (RCTs) and quasi experiments.
  - **Non-experimental methods** (where no intervention is given and populations are observed and compared to a control group), for example, cohort and case controlled studies, cross-sectional studies, questionnaires/surveys.
- **Qualitative research** (sometimes called **primary research**) of which there are many different approaches such as:
  - Grounded theory
  - Phenomenology
  - Ethnography
  - Action research
  - Some questionnaires include qualitative questions
- **Guidelines and policy** (if these are based on research evidence).

Systematic reviews and good quality literature reviews

Systematic reviews and good quality literature reviews are very useful as they aim to summarize **all** the available literature on a topic, either qualitative or quantitative. A literature review might be referred to as a **systematic review**, and this is the name given to a very detailed review of literature on a topic. The term 'systematic review' comes from the influence of the **Cochrane** and the **Campbell Collaboration** who commission literature reviews within health and social care. The Cochrane Collaboration is an organization which focusses on the commissioning and publication of systematic reviews within healthcare and the Campbell Collaboration focusses on reviews within a wider social care context. Both organizations specialize in the commissioning of high quality systematic reviews and if you come across a systematic review you can be fairly sure you have found a good quality review. Systematic literature reviews are referred to as original empirical research as they review, evaluate and synthesize all the available primary data, which can be either quantitative or qualitative.

A systematic review aims to identify and track down all the available literature on a topic with clear explanations of the approach taken.

Systematic reviews can be found in both health and social care topics and using any type of research. On both the Cochrane and Campbell Collaboration you can browse by topic for reviews and they have a plain English summary to help you understand complex medical or sociological terms or concepts.

Cochrane Library available at http://www.cochrane.org/reviews/
Campbell Library available at http://www.campbellcollaboration.org/

Cochrane states its vision as being '*that healthcare decision-making throughout the world will be informed by high-quality, timely research evidence*'.

  A less detailed review is often referred to as a **literature review** (that is *without* the prefix systematic). However, if the word 'systematic' is not found in the title, you might still have a high quality review – but you need to take a look at how the review was undertaken and you will form a judgement about the quality of the review.

How can I recognize a systematic review or a good literature review when I see one?

Most obviously of course, the title of the review will usually contain the words 'literature review' or 'systematic review'. However, the review itself will contain a written **method** which describes how the review has been undertaken. A systematic review or good quality literature review will tell you *how* the review was undertaken. If this is not explained, it is difficult to determine if the review has been carried out in a comprehensive manner and therefore how thorough it is. Information which should be included is how the reviewers searched for literature, and how they assessed the quality of what they included in their review.

Be wary of papers described as a 'literature review' or 'review' but which do not tell you how the review was compiled. The authors may have "cherry picked" what they wanted to include or ignored large areas of literature. There are lots of these 'review' papers in the literature and many are extremely useful, written by experts. However it is important to remember that unless they tell you how they searched and appraised the literature they included, it is not possible to tell whether the paper presents a balanced argument.

> **Example:** Linus Pauling (1986), the world accredited scientist, wrote a book entitled *How to Live Longer and Feel Better*, in which he quoted from a selection of articles that supported his opinion that vitamin C contains properties that are effective against the common cold. This book makes an interesting and convincing read. At first glance you might think it to be a comprehensive literature review, however no methodology was included in the book and, much later on, when a systematic review was undertaken of all the evidence surrounding the effectiveness of vitamin C, (Knipschild, 1994), no evidence of the effectiveness of vitamin C was identified. This illustrates how a non-systematic review can be misleading.

A systematic review or good quality literature review will be written up in the same manner as a research article; it should have:

- A clear research/review question
- Aims and objectives
- A methods section outlining how the review was undertaken
- A results section
- A discussion and conclusion.

 If the information you find does not contain a research question, aims and objectives, methods, results, discussion and conclusion then it is unlikely to be a thorough literature review.

Why are reviews so useful?

Literature reviews are important because they seek to:

- Summarize the literature that is available on any one topic
- Prevent one 'high profile' piece of information having too much influence
- Present an analysis of the available literature so that the reader does not have to access each individual research report included in the review.

It often seems to be the case that a piece of research is published one month which contradicts the findings of a piece of research published the month before. For example, one week we are told that alcohol has certain health benefits, the next week we are told that it is harmful. There is often confusion – people are trying to make sense of the differing messages conveyed and wonder why the results can vary so much. This can be due to:

- Looking at the results of a study in isolation rather than in the context of others
- Media portrayal of the research in which a complex set of results is reduced to a simplified message
- Not acknowledging that there are many aspects of health and social care; alcohol might have a positive effect on one aspect and a damaging effect on another.

An individual piece of health and social care information, taken in isolation, does not necessarily help the reader to achieve a better understanding of the bigger picture towards which the information contributes.

There are many reasons for this:

- The research might have been undertaken in a specific area of practice or with a specific group of people, or sample, and is not generalizable (or applicable) to other areas.
- There might be flaws in the research design which affect its overall usefulness.

Therefore when you read a report that seems to conflict with a report you read the previous week, it is important to consider the merits of each individual report and to remember that each single piece of research should not be viewed in isolation.

Try and notice examples of conflicting information in your own practice and then consider how much better it would be if all the information was togther so you could see the bigger picture.

Systematic reviews and literature reviews put the evidence into context.

They prevent one piece of evidence having excessive influence. One isolated piece of literature can be misleading. Take the story of the measles, mumps and rubella (MMR) vaccine. In 1998, Professor Wakefield and colleagues published an article in the *Lancet* suggesting that there was a possibility of a link between the MMR vaccination, autism and bowel disorders. This article was based on a small case study of twelve children, who had attended Wakefield's hospital, who had the conditions above and who had also had the vaccination. Wakefield stated that there were possible environmental triggers to the development of autism in these children, but without a control group and with a very small sample, this was very uncertain.

The paper published by Wakefield provided one piece of the jigsaw. At that time, there were no other data surrounding any potential link between autism and bowel disease. However, as time went on, many further studies were undertaken. No further studies confirmed any evidence of a link. It is easy to identify from the basic facts presented in the original paper that the evidence presented is not strong. Indeed the paper has subsequently been retracted by The *lancet* and the debate about the case continues unabated (Kmietowicz 2012) However, seen in isolation, this report sparked alarm in both media and medical circles alike. Systematic reviews and literature reviews help to shed new light.

The MMR controversy provides one clear example as to why it is important to review all the evidence together and how one piece of information can give a misleading picture. Without the comprehensive review of the literature which followed Wakefield's paper, the concerns expressed in his initial paper could not have been refuted. There are many similar examples in the literature, for example, in a Cochrane review by Farley *et al.* (2012), the role of a drug used to facilitate weight loss was reviewed. It had been previously thought that the use of drugs played only a minor role in weight loss facilitation programmes. On reviewing the available literature in a systematic way, the role of these drugs was found to be larger than had been thought.

Important points about a systematic review or good quality literature review

The following bullet points highlight the main features of a systematic review or a detailed literature review. At the end of each set of bullet points, we will give an example from a published systematic review in which this has been achieved.

- Reviewers should identify a clearly *pre-defined question.*
- Reviewers should undertake a *comprehensive* and *thorough search* for relevant literature, and should demonstrate how they have done this.
- Reviewers should search for *hard to find* articles including those that have not been published or not yet accepted for publication. This is because there is evidence that studies showing a positive result are more likely to be published – hence using only published studies could bias the result of the review.
- Researchers should develop *inclusion and exclusion criteria* in order to assess which information should be included in the review to ensure that only those papers that are relevant to the question(s) are included. Sometimes papers are given a grading according to pre-defined criteria and only the papers with a higher grading are included in the review.

Example: A systematic review carried out by Welsh and Farringdon (2008) explored the effectiveness of closed circuit television (CCTV) on the rates of crime. Given the importance of reviews in an evidence-based approach, we will discuss this example in detail. The question addressed by the review is clearly important as much public money is spent on CCTV and the extent to which they help to reduce crime is very relevant. The review is published by the Campbell Collaboration. Welsh and Farringdon document the method by which they undertook the review. Note in particular the way they undertook and document their search strategy:

Four search strategies were employed to identify studies meeting the criteria for inclusion in this review:

(1) searches of electronic bibliographic databases;
(2) searches of literature reviews on the effectiveness of CCTV in preventing crime;
(3) searches of bibliographies of CCTV studies; and
(4) contacts with leading researchers.

Both published and unpublished reports were considered in the searches. Searches were international in scope and were not limited to the English language.

(Welsh and Farringdon 2008: 2–3)

Once the reviewers have identified the range of literature to be included in the review, the next step is to assess the quality of the literature to see if it is good enough to help answer the question – using poor quality evidence may give us a misleading picture!

Researchers should *critique* (or judge) the quality of the selected papers to assess the quality of the research identified. Studies that do not meet the inclusion and quality criteria are excluded from the review. This is to ensure that only high quality and relevant papers are included.

We can look at how Welsh and Farringdon (2008) judged the quality of the studies they found for potential inclusion in their study:

For each study, we assessed methodological quality against one main characteristic: the presence of a reasonably comparable control area. In addition, the study had to report the number of crimes before and after in experimental and control areas.

(Welsh and Farringdon 2008: 7)

Finally reviewers *combine* the findings of all the papers that are used using a systematic approach. This enables new insights to be drawn from the summary of the papers that were not available before.

> If we look at Welsh and Farringdon's study we can see that the authors undertook a 'meta-analysis' of the results from different studies. A meta-analysis is a way of combining the results of different studies using statistics so that it is possible to merge the results of several studies, rather than having many different results from smaller studies.
>
> *A meta-analysis is carried out in order to estimate the average effect size in evaluations of the effects of CCTV on crime.*
>
> (Welsh and Farringdon 2008: 9)

It is important to note that a meta-analysis can only be carried out if all the research papers in the literature review have been undertaken in a similar way. And, as meta-analysis is a statistical technique, it can only be undertaken on papers that have their results presented as statistics. Where a meta-analysis has been undertaken, the results are often presented using a **forest plot**, in which the average result of each study is plotted so that it can be easily compared with other studies. As we will see later in this chapter, not all research papers present their results as statistics and for those which do not, it is not possible to do a meta-analysis. For these more qualitative papers, it is possible to combine the results which may be presented as themes, using a process known as **meta-synthesis** or **meta-study.**

> Welsh and Farringdon (2008: 3) concluded in the results of the study that:
>
> *The studies included in this systematic review indicate that CCTV has a modest but significant desirable effect on crime, is most effective in reducing crime in car parks, is most effective when targeted at vehicle crimes (largely a function of the successful car park schemes), and is more effective in reducing crime in the UK than in other countries.*

We can see from the results given above that they employed a robust search strategy to ensure a comprehensive approach to the inclusion of literature in their review. Their results were used to confirm the positive impact of CCTV.

Look on one of the sites for systematic reviews and find a topic relevant to your own professional practice that has been reviewed. See if it has all the components of a systematic review we have described.

Literature reviews (using less detailed approaches)

If you come across a literature review that is not specifically called a systematic review, this can still be a useful find if the review has been carried out in a systematic manner, even if not in the detail required by the Cochrane or Campbell Collaboration. What is important is to look at the method in which the review was undertaken, and make sure you can see a clear question, search strategy and a method of appraisal.

If you come across what you think might be a literature review but which has no clearly defined method or systematic approach, you should be less confident in the results of this review. These are sometimes referred to as narrative or descriptive reviews. In principle, you should be cautious about a literature review that:

- Has no focussed research question
- Has no detailed and complete searching strategy
- Has no clear method of appraisal or synthesis of literature
- Is not easily **repeatable.**

Consequently, the conclusions drawn are likely to be inaccurate. These reviews are likely to have a number of biases, including the personal bias of the author/s, as was evidence in Linus Pauling's book mentioned previously. If there is no clear method section, there is likely to be a bias in the selection of included material and conclusions, which cannot be easily verified and may therefore be misleading.

In summary, literature reviews are very useful as they consolidate the existing evidence on a topic. As a health and social care practitioner you cannot be expected to read, evaluate, assimilate and apply all the information on any one topic even if you could find it in the first place! However some literature reviews will be of a better quality than others; what is important is that you check out the way that the review has been written so that you can ensure that a comprehensive approach has been undertaken.

Quantitative research

Quantitative research seeks to quantify or measure the items under exploration in the study.

Quantitative research (sometimes called primary or positivist research) normally refers to studies which use methods of data collection that involve the use of numbers.

You will therefore find quantitative research when you are looking for research about topics that can be **measured numerically**, for example, how many people quitted smoking after a campaign, or how many people are satisfied with a particular service provided.

Some important points about quantitative research

- Quantitative research is undertaken only when data can be collected numerically.
- The studies tend to involve many participants and the findings can be applied in other contexts.
- Quantitative research often resembles a traditional experiment or study – there is no involvement between the researcher and participant (the aim is to be objective).
- Data are analysed using statistical tests.

Sampling

 Sample size in quantitative research tends to be large. This is because researchers are concerned with validity; that is, whether the findings of a study are valid or reflect reality.

For example, you are likely to have greater confidence in a study comparing two treatment options in which many thousands of people had participated than a study conducted on just twenty participants.

 Think of the last piece of research you have read. Consider how appropriate the sample size involved in the research was.

If the condition under investigation is unusual, sample sizes will inevitably be smaller. However paradoxically, you need to get big numbers in a study to be able to find out about the incidence rate.

Quantitative studies often use random sampling and/or random allocation – these two terms are often confused and it is important to recognize the difference between the two.

Random sampling is defined as meaning that all those in the sample have an equal chance of being selected in the sample. This ensures that the sample is not biased. Compare this to **convenience sampling,** which as its name suggests, is where the sample is taken from participants who are local or otherwise 'convenient' to the study.

An example: A random sample of university students could be drawn from the university admission lists rather than from the attendance at lectures, given that all students will be on the admission list, but not all will attend lectures. Any sample drawn from those who attend lectures will be biased rather than random. It is important to note that obtaining an unbiased sample in any research study is very difficult. A questionnaire might be sent to a random sample of the population, but unless there is a 100 per cent **response rate,** the responses obtained will be biased.

Contrast this with **random allocation;** which is where the sample is not random but participants within a non random sample (for example a convenience sample) are allocated at random into one group or another. Random allocation is used within an RCT where those involved in the study are not selected at random but are allocated at random to one group within the study. We discuss this in more detail further on in this chapter.

Experimental and non-experimental quantitative research

Quantitative research can be divided into experimental and non-experimental research.

Experimental methods can be used to measure the effectiveness of an intervention (for example, smoking cessation interventions). In this case, quantitative methods could be used to compare how many people give up smoking in the intervention group and in the non-intervention group. This would be measured numerically, in months and years. The important thing here is that the experimenter controls who has what intervention. Hence we call it an experiment. There are **non-experimental** research designs, such as questionnaires/surveys in which participants respond to questions. Their responses can then be counted numerically – for example 30 per cent of those who responded to the survey had done X.

In principle quantitative research is generally undertaken when you are looking to measure something and that something is suitable for numerical measurement. Let's look in more detail at some of the quantitative research designs that you are likely to encounter.

Types of experimental quantitative studies

We will discuss the experimental quantitative studies you may come across, starting with the randomized controlled trial (RCT). It is an important design and once you have understood the basic principles of an RCT, you can see more easily how the other quantitative studies work.

Randomized Controlled Trials

Randomized controlled trials are a form of clinical trial, or scientific procedure used to determine the effectiveness of a treatment, intervention or medicine.

RCTs are useful when you are looking to find out **whether a treatment or intervention is effective or better than an alternative intervention.** In this case, you should search for RCTs in the first instance. If you find some RCTs, then you probably have good evidence about the effectiveness of your treatment or intervention. If you do not find any RCTs or a review of RCTS then you cannot answer your question regarding whether the intervention or therapy works or not.

Some important points about an RCT

- It is widely considered to be the most thorough ('gold standard') form of evidence when we are considering whether a treatment or intervention is effective.
- In an RCT, participants are allocated by random allocation into two or more groups.
- An intervention is then given to one of the groups and not given to the other (control) group; the outcome of the two groups is then compared.
- If it is not possible to randomize participants in a research study and expose one group to a particular intervention (for example, for ethical reasons) then it is not possible to carry out an RCT.

An example: The practice of swaddling babies used to be very common in many cultures and is maintained today in very cold climates. This practice was (and is) necessary to protect babies from the severe cold and as a means of keeping babies safe during travel. However as times developed and different options became available for protecting children, the question of whether the practice of swaddling is harmful to babies has become significant. For this reason a team of researchers, Manaseki-Holland *et al.* (2010) undertook a randomized controlled trial to find out if swaddling babies has any negative effect on the babies' growth and development. The researchers described the trial:

> *1279 healthy new-borns in Ulaanbaatar, Mongolia, were allocated at birth to traditional swaddling or non-swaddling. The families received 7 months of home visits to collect data and monitor compliance. At 11 to 17 months of age, (the trial) was administered to 1100 children.*
> (Manaseki-Holland *et al.* 2010)

Randomized controlled trials are generally considered to be the best way (and many people would say the only way) to determine whether a new treatment or intervention is effective or an established treatment is harmful or not. In the above example, the intervention investigated was the introduction of clothing and the control group was the standard practice of swaddling newborn babies.

The importance of randomization

Participants are allocated into the different treatment groups of the trial at **random**. This is like the tossing of a coin. This ensures that participants are allocated into the different groups by chance rather than by the preference of the patient/client or researcher. It is very important that neither the participant nor the researcher has any control over the group to which a participant is allocated.

Example continued . . .

If we take the Mongolian study, the process of randomization required that mothers of the babies did not have any input into which group their babies were entered into. One group were allocated to the traditional practice of swaddling whilst the other group were given extra warm layers of clothing. It must have been quite daunting for the mothers of the babies in the intervention group who were not swaddled but were dressed in extra layers of clothing, to go against years of traditional practice! When they agreed to participate in the study, they were informed that their baby could be allocated to either of the two groups.

Randomization is important because there need to be equal groups. This is because the researcher is looking for differences between the treatment group and the control group. If the groups are random, then any differences in outcome can be said to be due to the intervention. This can only be determined if the different groups, which are commonly referred to as 'arms', of the trial are essentially equal in all respects except for the treatment given. The researcher is looking for differences between the different groups of the trial that can be attributed to the intervention.

> **Example continued . . .**
>
> In the case of the Mongolian babies, researchers were looking to see if the practice of swaddling had any effect on the babies' development, when this group of babies were compared to babies who had not been swaddled.

Why can't participants choose which group they want to go into?

If the research participants were allowed to choose which group of the RCT they wanted to enter, it is very likely that one particular treatment group would be more popular than another, although it's not always possible to say which. This would mean that the different groups in the trial would not be equal.

Without equal groups, it is not be possible to determine whether the differences in outcomes observed between the different treatment or control groups of the trial were due to the intervention or whether they were due to the differences in the characteristics of the participants who had self-selected into one group or another.

Do the groups in an RCT have similar characteristics after randomization?

The randomization process normally results in the creation of equal groups. If it is particularly important that participants with specific characteristics are equally represented in both groups (for example, those in certain age groups or those who care for relatives might have different lifestyle habits from those without children and you might want an equal number of these participants in each group) then a further form of randomization can be used. This is an additional statistical process that assists in ensuring that the groups are equal in respect of certain predefined criteria (for example age, sex, or smoker) that are relevant for the research, and it is called stratification or minimization.

 Can you explain the difference between random sampling and randomization?

How does an RCT work?

Once each treatment group in the trial has been randomly allocated, the groups are considered to be equal, and the intervention, treatment or therapy is given to the first group. This is often called the 'independent variable'. The second group receives either the standard treatment (or no treatment or placebo, depending on the individual study design). The groups are then observed and the differences between the groups are monitored. Given that the two groups of participants were randomly allocated and hence can be considered to be 'equal', any difference between the groups can be attributed to the effect of the intervention. The outcome measured is often called the 'dependent variable'

The **non-intervention** group may be:

- **A control group** who receive the established **standard treatment or intervention** *(while the intervention group receive the new treatment/intervention).*
- **A placebo group** who receive a dummy drug or sham treatment, but the important thing is that the participants do not know this! If at all possible, neither the researcher running the trial nor the participants know which group they have been allocated to. A placebo group is however only **ethical** if non-treatment is not thought to be harmful to participants – let's say if there was genuine uncertainty as to the effectiveness of a treatment.

This is called **blinding** and a study can either be **double blind** – when neither the researcher nor participants know which group the participants are in, or **single blind** – when the researchers only know which group the participants are in. This obviously depends on what the study is looking for and whether it is possible to blind either the researchers or participants.

Example continued . . .

In the Mongolian study, there was a control group, who were the group of babies given the traditional practice of swaddling. The intervention group were given extra layers of clothing. At the end of the trial, researchers look to see what the differences in outcome are between the different groups in the trial – for example, what was the difference in growth and development between the babies who had been swaddled and those who had not? Because the groups were otherwise equal, we can say that any difference in outcome is likely to be attributable to the intervention versus control (clothing versus swaddling).

Why do we have a 'null' hypothesis?

A null hypothesis is usually stated when an RCT is designed. The null hypothesis is a starting point – it is a 'negatively' phrased statement that asserts that *there is no difference between the two groups*. The aim of the RCT is to determine whether this assertion, i.e. the null hypothesis, can be confirmed or rejected. If the results show that there is a difference between the control group and the intervention group, then the null hypothesis can be rejected.

Example continued . . .

In the Mongolian study, researchers described the null hypothesis as follows:

The null hypothesis was that Mongolian infants not swaddled or swad-dled tightly in a traditional setting (to >7 months of age) do not have sig-nificantly different scores for the Bayley Scales of Infant Development, Second Edition (BSID-II).

(Manaseki-Holland *et al.* 2010)

A flow diagram of the process of conducting an RCT for the Mongolian study babies is presented below:

Newborn babies were recruited in a clinic in Ulaanbaata, Mongolia.

⇓

Mothers of the babies who agreed to participate in the study were informed about the process of randomization. This population was then randomly allocated into two groups:

⇓

1 Group One babies carry on normal swaddling practice.
2 Group Two babies receive additional clothing but are not swaddled.

⇓

The rate and range of movement and overall development of the babies in the different groups is then compared at set points in the study. Any differences in outcomes are attributed to the swaddling or non-swaddling, given that the groups were random-ized and therefore otherwise equal.

In the Mongolian study, the researchers found that there were no differences in the growth and development of the babies in either group. They described their results as follows. (Note the term 'significant' is a statistical term which we discuss later in this chapter.)

No significant between-group differences were found in mean scaled mental and psychomotor developmental scores.

(Manaseki-Holland *et al.* 2010)

The Mongolian swaddling study illustrates how the RCT can be used to deter-mine whether an intervention is beneficial or harmful.

Differences between the two or more groups in an RCT are often expressed as a **risk ratio or odds ratio.** To understand these terms, consider a study that explored the effect of a new intervention to help people stop smoking. In the intervention group, 40 out of 100 people stop smoking. In the control group, only 20 out of 100 people stop smoking. To calculate how much more likely you are to stop smoking if you take the new intervention, we take the proportion of people who stop with the new drug (40/100) and divide by the proportion of people in the control group who stop (20/100). The answer is 2 and we can say that people are twice as likely to stop smoking if they use the intervention. This figure is the risk ratio. The odds ratio is slightly less intuitive and is not often used for reporting trials and is defined in the glossary. RCTs can only be used when it is possible to allocate participants within a group at random and administer a treatment or intervention to one group and not to the other. When this cannot be done, often for ethical reasons, a modified experiment may be considered.

Quasi experiments

Quasi experiments are experiments which have some of the features of an RCT but not all of them. They are usually carried out when it is not possible to undertake a RCT.

> **For example:** if you were exploring infant nutrition, it would not be acceptable or ethical to ask one group of mothers to abstain from breastfeeding their babies in order to make a comparison with another group of mothers who were asked to breastfeed.

Quasi experiments are most useful when you need to find out if something is effective, but are not able to undertake a randomized controlled trial.

The important point about a quasi experiment is that they share many of the same characteristics as a RCT. They deviate from this design usually when circumstances demand that adherence to the RCT method is not practical or ethical.

> **For example:** Imagine you want to find out whether a new style of parenting class is effective. Because of the nature of childcare, it is not possible to undertake an RCT. Instead you implement the new style of class with one group of parents who have enrolled on a parenting class and compare the

results with another group in another area who have not completed this class. You can see that the two groups in the experiment are not equal – the parents in one class might come from different sociological groups than those in another and whilst you might allow for this by selecting similar areas to take part in the study, you will not achieve equal groups as you would in an RCT. Therefore if the outcomes for the parents who experienced the new style of parenting class were different from the outcomes of those who did not, you cannot tell if these outcomes would be different due to other factors.

Therefore in a quasi experiment, it is not possible to say with as much certainty that the outcome was due to the intervention administered. Whilst non-randomized experiments will provide you with evidence, this is generally thought to be **second best evidence** if you are looking to determine the evidence of effectiveness.

Non-experimental quantitative methods

Cohort studies and case control studies are studies that try to link up the causes of diseases and/or interventions and/or social situations. Cohort studies and case control studies were first used to observe the effects of an exposure (say smoking) on the health of those observed.

Cohort and case control studies are most useful when you need information about the likely causes of disease and other problems but you are not able to do an experiment. For example, you wonder whether excessive alcohol leads to dementia. Of course you cannot do an experiment to find this out but you can follow up those who do drink and compare the rate of dementia with those who do not.

Some important points about cohort and case control studies

- They have been used most often to find the causes or impact of disease.
- They are then followed up in order to observe the effect of the exposure to – for example – smoking nicotine, on the health and social wellbeing of those observed.

 Cohort studies are observational studies. These studies attempt to discover the causes of disease or problem when it is not possible to carry out an experiment.

A cohort study is the study of a group of people who have all been exposed to a particular event or lifestyle (for example let's say that they all smoke, or have a particular disability).

For example: A cohort study published by Allen *et al.* in 2009 was able to identify that women who drink even modest amounts of alcohol are more at risk of developing breast cancer than their non-drinking counterparts. Women attending a clinic for breast cancer screening were followed up and the drinking habits of those who went on to develop breast cancer were compared to those who did not develop the disease.

This is how the cohort study was described:

The Million Women Study has been described previously. In 1996–2001 a total of 1.3 million middle-aged women who attended breast cancer screening clinics in the United Kingdom completed a questionnaire that asked for socio-demographic and other personal information, including how much wine, beer, and spirits they drank on average each week. Information on whether the wine consumed was red, white or both was also recorded. In a follow-up survey, done about 3 years after recruitment, study participants were again asked to report the usual number of alcoholic drinks consumed per week.

(Allen *et al.* 2009)

This cohort study demonstrated that there was a strong association between alcohol consumption and development of breast cancer.

A flow diagram of the process of conducting a cohort study:

Cohort of people who all experienced the same exposure/experience.

⇓

This cohort is followed up to observe the effect of this exposure.

They may be compared to the control group who did not experience this exposure, but because the groups were not formed by random allocation, any observed differences between the two groups at the end of the study period are not as easily attributable to the exposure as if the study had been an RCT.

A case control study works the other way round to a cohort study. People (cases) that have a condition are studied and compared to cases that do not. You could for example explore the alcohol consumption of those who have developed breast cancer and compare this against those who do not have the disease.

A case control study is one in which patient/clients with a particular condition are studied and *compared with* others who do not have that condition in order to try to establish whether a particular exposure has led to a condition.

Example: In 1954, Doll and Hill carried out a case control study examining lung cancer. In their study, patients/clients were traced back to see what could have caused the disease. They designed a questionnaire which was given to patients/clients with suspected lung, liver or bowel cancer. Those administering the questionnaire were not aware which of the diseases was suspected in which patients/clients. It became clear from the questionnaires that those who were later confirmed to have lung cancer were also confirmed smokers. Those who did not have lung cancer did not smoke. Clearly it would not have been ethical to have undertaken an RCT to explore the causes of lung cancer as it would not have been possible to randomize a group of non-smokers and ask one group to start smoking!

A flow diagram of the process of conducting a case control study:

Individuals with a specific condition or situation are identified.

⇓

The circumstances that led up to the development/progress of this condition are then explored.

Questionnaire/surveys/cross-sectional studies

Questionnaires and surveys are a popular type of (usually) quantitative research which you have probably been involved with yourself on many occasions. They provide a snapshot of participants' responses to questions on a particular topic at a given point in time.

Questionnaire/surveys are studies in which a sample is taken at any one point in time (cross-section of a population) from a defined group of people and observed/assessed.

Questionnaire/surveys are most useful when you are looking for evidence about frequency of a particular activity, or information about a large group of people. Remember that questionnaire/survey studies have many limitations as outlined below and the results of these should be viewed with caution.

Some important points about questionnaires

- Questionnaires can be used to collect data in RCTs, cohort and case control studies.
- Questionnaires which are poorly designed will lead to misleading conclusions!
- A questionnaire will only collect useful data if the questions have been well tested and piloted.
- A long questionnaire might be discarded before completion.
- Complicated or badly worded questions may be misunderstood by the respondent.
- Postal questionnaires have the additional disadvantage that there is likely to be a low response rate.
- If large sections of the target population do not respond, the overall quality of data that is collected will be poor.
- It is often not possible to get access to a fully representative sample for the distribution of a questionnaire.
- The completed questionnaires will contain information from a selection of, but not a random sample of, participants and will therefore give an incomplete picture of the target population.
- Any apparent associations arising from the analysis of questionnaire data should be interpreted with caution.

For example: if it was identified that those who used illicit drugs also experienced high anxiety levels, it would be tempting to conclude that use of illicit drugs increases student anxiety. However perhaps the reverse is true and those with high levels of anxiety resort to illicit drug use.

For example: if you distributed the questionnaire in a shopping centre on a Saturday, you would reach a different population than if the questionnaire was distributed on a weekday. Similarly, you would be likely to get a different group of people depending on the time at which the questionnaire was distributed. Distributing the questionnaire on different days of the week at different times would help to alleviate this.

Data analysis in quantitative research

There are two main types of statistics: *descriptive and inferential.*

Descriptive statistics describe the data given in the paper. These statistics should clearly describe the main results, for example how many people answered 'yes' to a particular question or what the most common response to a question was.

The results will typically be given as follows:

- **Mean:** this is the average when all the results are added up and divided by the number of participants. **Example:** if results from 5 participants were 25, 35, 20, 20, 40 then the average score would be the total of this (140) divided by the number of participants (5) (= an average score of 28).
- **Median:** the middle value if the results are ranked from lowest to highest.
- **Example:** in 11 results as follows 1, 1, 2, 3, 3, **4**, 5, 6, 6, 7, 7 the number 4 is in the middle.
- **Mode:** this is the number that occurs most often so in 1, 1, 2, **3**, **3**, **3**, 6, 7, 8, 8, then 3 is the mode as it occurs three times.
- **Percentages** are also used. This indicates how many out of 100 such as 65 out of 100 = 65%.
- **Standard deviation:** shows how much deviation from the mean.

Inferential statistics generalize to the wider population. In other words, to determine the extent to which the results obtained from the sample in the research have any relevance to the **wider population** as a whole.

- Inferential statistics do more than describe a sample, they infer or predict how likely that is to apply to the wider population.
- The bigger the sample, the surer you can be that the sample prevalence is close to the population prevalence.

Example: At the time of a general election, opinion polls are used to predict the overall result of the election. These polls are based on a small sample of voters but are used with good accuracy to predict the overall result.

Confidence intervals

You might see two numbers written besides the main findings or results in a bracket. These are called confidence intervals and this is what they mean:

Imagine you want to know how many people are going to vote for the Green Party. If you asked 10 people and two people told you they were going to vote for this party, you would be fairly uncertain about how the voting was likely to go but if you asked 100 people and 20 people told you they were going to vote for the Green Party you would have more of an idea. If you asked 1000 people and 200 were going to vote for the Green Party, you would have a more precise prediction. In each case you are drawing a sample of the electorate to predict how the whole electorate or population is going to vote. In research we take a sample in order to make a general rule of what is true of the whole population.

Confidence intervals express the uncertainty of our estimate.

Thinking of the examples above, the first sample of 10 people would have more uncertainty than the third example in which 1000 people were consulted. This is expressed in a confidence interval which quantifies the uncertainty. So if two people out of 10 told you they were going to vote for the green party, the confidence intervals would likely to be wide. The best estimate would be that 20% people of the population would vote for the Green party but you would not be very certain about this and would express that uncertainty by giving a range of percentages of people who might vote Green–for example 4–56%. This means that we can be 95% sure that somewhere between 4% and 56% of the population will vote for the Green Party. In the example where 1000 people were consulted, again the best estimate would be that 20% would vote for the Green Party but because the sample is larger, the confidence intervals would be smaller – for example 18–23%. This means that we can be 95% certain that somewhere between 18 and 23% of the population will vote Green. Confidence intervals are worked out using a statistical formula and are calculated with a 95% confidence interval. This means that we can be 95% sure that the confidence intervals are between the ranges stated.

- The smaller the interval or range, the more confident you can be that the results in the study reflect the results you would find in the larger population.
- Using a formula, the confidence intervals, upper and lower are calculated. A **95% confidence interval** means that we can be 95% sure that the true population prevalence lies between the lower and upper confidence interval.

Probability value (p value)

Statistics are often described as a *p value* or probability value. The p value expresses the probability of the difference shown between the groups in an experiment being due to chance. It is important to determine the likelihood that the findings are down to chance in any research.

The lower the p value the less likely it is that the occurrence is due to chance. If a p value is less than 0.05 (1:20) we say the occurrence is unlikely to be due to chance. If the p value is much less that 0.05 (1:20) for example p = 0.005 (1:200) then the occurrence is even more unlikely to be due to chance.

Example: You are undertaking an RCT comparing different ways to help people stop smoking. Normally in an RCT, you would give an intervention to one group and not to the other and then examine the differences in outcomes between the groups.

However if both groups were treated with the standard treatment you would likely see a variety of outcomes in each group due to natural differences between the groups. Then, you administer an intervention to one of the groups and observe the different outcomes of the two groups. The p value can then be calculated to determine whether the differences in outcomes observed is due to chance or not.

To calculate the p value we refer to the **null hypothesis.** In the philosophy of science, we can never prove something is true, we can only disprove. For this reason, we develop a hypothesis which is the opposite of what we actually believe – this is the null hypothesis. This is a phrase that is used when you state (in order to test it), that there is no relationship between the different elements (or **variables**) under study. For example *'there is no difference in outcomes for parents who attend parenting classes and those who do not.'* This hypothesis can be tested using the results from the study when the different groups are compared and calculated using a statistical test, such as the Chi squared test. A p value of 0.05, for example, means there is a (1:20) chance of seeing these results if the null hypothesis were true. So, this means that there is a relationship between the variables. It is important to remember that this does not indicate a causal relationship, i.e. that one variable caused the other, but just that the two occur together.

This basic outline of some of the statistics you might come across is to help you understand how statistics are used to tell us about the strength of the results we are looking at. They help us to understand if a particular piece of research helps us to answer a question. Next time you read a paper with statistics in, ask yourself what the statistics say about the results and the strength of evidence presented.

Qualitative studies

Qualitative studies typically **do not seek to quantify or measure** the items under exploration using numbers as in quantitative research. Instead they aim to explore an issue in depth. They are often carried out on an area or topic where little is known.

The principle of all qualitative approaches is to explore the meaning of and *develop in-depth understanding* of the research topic as experienced by the participants of the research.

The results of qualitative research are not expressed in percentages and numbers but as **words** in the form of **descriptive themes.**

Qualitative research is most useful when you are looking for in-depth insight or answers to questions that cannot be answered numerically, when you are asking why? or how? or what?

Think of an area of your own practice where you could explore a qualitative question relating to the experience, or understanding, of an issue.

Some important points about qualitative studies

- This research is sometimes referred to as naturalistic research.
- Researchers seek to understand the *whole* of an experience and insight of the situation.
- The data collected is not numerical but is collected, often through interview, using the words and descriptions given by participants.
- There is no use of statistics in qualitative research; the results are **descriptive** and **interpretative.**
- They do not set out looking for specific ideas, hoping to confirm pre-existing beliefs. Instead, they code the data and build themes according to ideas arising from within it. This process is often referred to as **inductive.**
- The generation of themes, although rigorous, is **interpretative and subjective**, depending on the insight of the researcher.
- The researcher cannot achieve complete objectivity because he or she is the data collection tool (for example, the interviewer) and subjectively interprets the data that is collected. This is acknowledged in the research process and steps are taken to maintain credibility and trustworthiness in this process as far as possible.
- Sample sizes tend to be small. A small sample is required because in-depth understanding (rather than statistical analysis) is sought from information-rich participants who take part.
- The **participants used** in a qualitative study tend not to be selected at random, instead participants are selected if they have had exposure to or experience of the phenomenon of interest in the particular study.
- This type of sampling is referred to as **purposive sampling** and this leads to the selection of information-rich cases who can contribute to the answering of the research question. Other approaches to sampling in qualitative research are **theoretical** – where the sample is determined according to

the needs of the study, and snowball sampling – where the sample is developed as new potential participants are identified as the study progresses. *For **example**, the contacts of participants already involved in the research may be invited to enter the study, if they have the relevant experience.*

 Large numbers of participants are rarely used (and are not necessarily appropriate) in qualitative research.

The richness of qualitative data arises from **the dialogue between the researcher and the researched** and the insights obtained through this process are only possible because of the **interaction** between the two. For example, the interviewer may probe the interviewee about his or her responses to a question and phrase the next question as a direct response to the reply received. **Subjectivity is required** for the researcher to get an insight into the topic of investigation and objectivity is not strived for.

Qualitative data analysis is **open to interpretation.** Because the researcher is involved in, and indeed shapes, both the data collection and analysis process, it is not possible for the researcher to remain detached from the data which is collected. The concept of **reflexivity** refers to the acknowledgement by the qualitative researcher that this process of enquiry is necessarily open to interpretation and that **detachment** from the focus of the research is **neither desirable nor possible.**

Examples of qualitative research questions

• What it is like for a patient/client who has had a stroke?
• What is the lived experience of mothers forced to leave their home due to repossession?
• How do patient/clients with newly diagnosed diabetes cope with their condition?
• Why do independent nurse prescribers prescribe less than general practitioners?

Different approaches to qualitative research

The most commonly used **data collection methods** in qualitative research are:

• In-depth interviews
• Focus groups
• Questionnaires using open-ended questions.

There are a wide variety of approaches to qualitative research. You are likely to encounter many different approaches when you read the literature. Some are just described in the literature as 'qualitative studies' whilst others are named according to the particular qualitative approach that is followed. These are outlined below. It is useful to recognize these different approaches and to understand why one approach was selected for a specific research question.

Grounded theory is a way of finding out about what happens in a social setting and then making wider generalizations about the way things happen. The purpose of grounded theory is to generate a theory from the data and observations that are made. It is a 'bottom up' approach in which data is collected and analysed and then used to make explanations about the way things happen in social life.

Grounded theory is most useful when you want to explore an area which has not been extensively studied and you are looking to develop theory about what is happening in a particular context.

For example: Mangnall and Yurkovich (2010) undertook a grounded theory study in order to explore (and develop a theory about) why women prisoners self harm. They undertook interviews and observations to explore when and why women self harm and concluded that self harm was a mechanism by which women released anger and anxiety. Yet this relief of anxiety was soon replaced by negative consequences of the punishment that followed self harm and hence a negative cycle was instigated. The researchers concluded that practitioners working in detention centres should allow the women to express their anxieties verbally without fear of reprisals.

Phenomenology is the study of the 'lived experience' or what it is actually like to live with a particular condition or experience. These studies often use in-depth interviews as the means of data collection as they allow the participant the opportunity to explore and describe their experience within an interview setting.

Phenomenology is most useful when you want to find out about individual experiences of an illness, social situation or event.

For example: Tebbet and Kennedy (2012) did a phenomenological study that explored the experience of childbirth for women with spinal cord injuries. They interviewed eight women about their experiences and from the analysis of these interviews were able to identify common themes. They found that despite the difficulties these women were facing, and contrary to popular belief, most women had a positive experience of childbirth and with individualized care were able to overcome difficulties caused by their condition.

Ethnography is the study of human culture. An ethnographic study focusses on a community (i.e. a specific group of people) in order to gain insight about how its members behave. Observation or participant observation and/or in-depth interviews may be undertaken to achieve this. As it seeks to observe phenomena as they occur in real time a true ethnographic study is a time consuming process.

Ethnography is most useful when you want to find out about a culture or way of life of a group of people in order to understand why they act and behave the way that they do.

For example: Ericsson *et al.* (2011) did an ethnographical study that explored how people with dementia interact within a care home for the elderly. The researchers undertook observations and interviews with residents in a home for elderly people. By observing and finding out about the everyday life of the residents with dementia, and their interactions with others, they found that those with dementia were often able to interact with others and had an awareness of their situation and surroundings, emphasizing the need to encourage interaction between all residents within a residential setting.

Action research is the process by which practitioners or researchers work together to address issues that arise in everyday practice in order to develop a systematic approach to change implementation and the evaluation of change. Action research is a cyclical method of planning, implementing and evaluating change and development in the working environment. Action research is often designed and conducted by practitioners who analyse the data to improve their own practice.

Action research is useful when you need to generate improvements in organizations that are not in the form of research findings, but are generated as solutions from within.

For example: Elliott (2003) explored the use of portfolios in an action research project designed to look at the development of continuing professional development within a social care setting. Changes in the use of the portfolio as a tool for continuing professional development were introduced and evaluated in the action research project.

You may also come across **discourse analysis,** which is an approach which analyses the use of language in order to understand meaning in complex areas. There are various approaches to this method (Hodges 2008).

Discourse analysis is most useful when the researcher wants to gain understanding of complex phenomena. Using analysis of the language people use in day-to-day communication helps to determine the reality of their beliefs and values rather than what they might say if asked questions or for their opinions.

> **For example:** Schofield *et al.* (2011) carried out a discourse analysis of how nurses understand and care for older people with delirium in the acute hospital – they found that the main focus of nurses was on surveillance and containment.

After reading this section, try and summarize your learning on literature reviews, quantitative and qualitative research methodologies. If you are unclear, read the section again or discuss it with a colleague or fellow student.

Which type of research is best?

There has been much debate in the research literature about the merits of different approaches to research (i.e. quantitative or qualitative) with some researchers claiming that one is better than another. In this book we argue that these debates are not important. This is because quantitative and qualitative approaches look at different things, or different aspects of the same problem; it is not possible or helpful to say that one is better than the other. There are many similarities between both approaches to research. Both commence with a research question and select the appropriate methodology to answer this question. In all research papers, the methods used to undertake the research should be clearly explained and the results clearly presented. This is known as **the research process** and is the same process as used to describe a systematic review or a primary research paper.

The most important thing is that the most *appropriate research methodology is used* to address what you need to find out.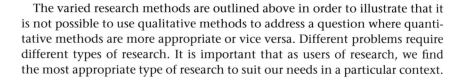

The varied research methods are outlined above in order to illustrate that it is not possible to use qualitative methods to address a question where quantitative methods are more appropriate or vice versa. Different problems require different types of research. It is important that as users of research, we find the most appropriate type of research to suit our needs in a particular context.

What does the term 'hierarchy of evidence' mean?

There is general agreement that a 'hierarchy of evidence' exists – that is, that *research can be ranked in order of importance* and that some forms of research evidence are stronger than others in addressing some types of research questions.

However, as you can deduce from the previous discussion, there is **no one single hierarchy of evidence.** There are different hierarchies depending on what you need to find out.

The 'traditional' hierarchy of evidence for determining effective treatment puts systematic reviews and randomized controlled trials at the top and qualitative studies at the bottom as shown below (Sackett *et al.* 1996).

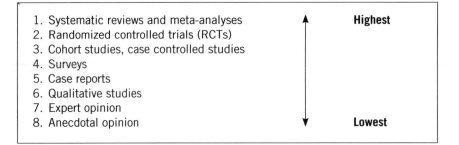

1. Systematic reviews and meta-analyses   **Highest**
2. Randomized controlled trials (RCTs)
3. Cohort studies, case controlled studies
4. Surveys
5. Case reports
6. Qualitative studies
7. Expert opinion
8. Anecdotal opinion   **Lowest**

In order to make sense of this hierarchy, first of all we need to acknowledge that (systematic) **literature reviews are almost always the strongest evidence.** Therefore most people would agree that a review should always be at the top of any hierarchy. So *position 1* in the hierarchy is not really in debate. However if we go to *position 2*, the second ranked item is the RCT, and this is where it gets more interesting. In the hierarchy of evidence above, the RCT is the next best form of evidence in the absence of a (systematic) literature review. This might be the case **IF** the research question you are interested in can be answered using an RCT, for example if you need to find out about the effectiveness of one intervention or treatment over another. Moving down to *positions 3–8*, further different types of evidence are given, with qualitative studies and expert opinion very low down in the ranking.

Can you identify the limitations of this type of hierarchy?

The limitation of this type of hierarchy is that it is **only** relevant if you are looking for evidence to determine whether a treatment or intervention is effective or not and therefore answerable using an RCT or review of RCTs as the best available evidence. We have seen earlier in this chapter how many research questions are not best addressed using RCTs or even quantitative studies at all. For these questions which are not answered by an RCT, this hierarchy is clearly not appropriate. It can therefore be misleading to consider just one hierarchy of evidence. In fact, what we really need are several hierarchies, which suit the different research questions we are likely to come across.

Determining your own hierarchy of evidence

We have emphasized throughout this book that it is important that you work out what type of information you need and you should seek this information in the first instance. If you need to find out if something works, then the 'traditional' hierarchy of evidence will work and you will be looking for RCTs (after reviews of RCTs) in the first instance. If your question is not about whether or not an intervention or therapy works, then you need to think more broadly for the type of evidence you need. In a previous publication, Aveyard (2010) refers to **developing your own 'hierarchy of evidence'** that you need to address the particular research question you are interested in. Noyes (2010) argues from a similar position and points out that different forms of evidence are valuable in particular contexts. There will be some contexts when qualitative research is more useful than quantitative research – for example if you want to know about patient or client experience so that a service can be improved. In these cases, qualitative research would be in *position 2* rather than *position 6* and the RCT would be somewhat lower ranked, if it appeared at all!

Noyes (2010: 530) gives an example of a hierarchy of evidence that could help us understand client or patient experience. The hierarchy of **'views and experiences of interventions and services'** is given below:

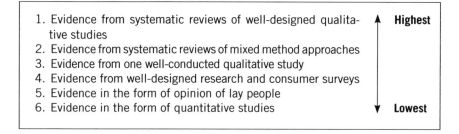

1. Evidence from systematic reviews of well-designed qualitative studies — **Highest**
2. Evidence from systematic reviews of mixed method approaches
3. Evidence from one well-conducted qualitative study
4. Evidence from well-designed research and consumer surveys
5. Evidence in the form of opinion of lay people
6. Evidence in the form of quantitative studies — **Lowest**

Noyes' (2010) hierarchy works well for research questions that are looking at qualitative experiences researched using qualitative methods and might be useful for the following question: *What is it like to enter the UK as a migrant worker?* If you want to find out what it is like to enter the UK as a migrant worker, you would need to find evidence of the experience of those workers. Therefore, qualitative studies, probably using a phenomenological account, would be at the top of your hierarchy of evidence.

However there are other research questions for which neither the 'traditional' or the 'views and experiences' hierarchies would be helpful. For example, let's say you are a public health specialist and need to find out whether people who have taken a particular drug are more at risk of a particular condition. Let's take for example thalidomide which was prescribed in the 1960s to pregnant women as an anti-sickness medication and which was found to lead to malformations in the babies of women who took the drug. In this case an RCT would not be appropriate as it would not be ethical to randomly allocate participants to receive either thalidomide or a placebo once you already had suspicions about a particular drug. Instead you would need to look for other types of quantitative studies – case controlled trials or cohort studies which explore the effects of a particular exposure on the population in question. Therefore cohort studies or case control studies would be at the top of the hierarchy in this instance of the evidence you are looking for.

The hierarchy of evidence (adapted from Noyes 2010) for **determining whether something works or not when you cannot undertake an RCT:**

1. Evidence from systematic reviews of well-designed cohort   ▲   **Highest**
   and case controlled studies
2. Evidence from systematic reviews of mixed method approaches
3. Evidence from one well-conducted cohort or case control study
4. Evidence from qualitative studies
5. Evidence in the form of opinion of lay people   ▼   **Lowest**

Let's take anther example. Imagine you want to find out whether public sector workers wash their hands prior to contact with their clients or patients. You would need to find evidence of what happens in practice by descriptions of care undertaken, or better still of observations of the care delivered. Therefore studies of observation of or accounts of care delivery would be at the top of your hierarchy of evidence in this instance.

The hierarchy of evidence (adapted from Noyes 2010) for **determining whether public sector workers wash their hands:**

1. Evidence from systematic reviews of well-designed observa-   ▲   **Highest**
   tional studies
2. Evidence from systematic reviews of mixed method approaches
3. Evidence from one well-conducted observational study
4. Evidence from qualitative studies
5. Evidence in the form of opinion of lay people   ▼   **Lowest**

As a final example in this section, imagine you wanted to find out how many students use illicit drugs whilst at university. You would need to find questionnaires/surveys which have explored this aspect of student life. Whilst the data collected from questionnaires can be unreliable, in this instance, there is really no other way to get at this data. Therefore, this data would be at the top of your hierarchy of evidence.

The hierarchy of evidence (adapted from Noyes 2010) for **identifying prevalence of drug use within a university population.**

---

1. Evidence from systematic reviews of well-designed questionnaire studies   ▲ **Highest**
2. Evidence from systematic reviews of mixed method approaches
3. Evidence from one well-conducted questionnaire study
4. Evidence from well-designed qualitative studies
5. Evidence in the form of opinion of lay people   ▼ **Lowest**

It should be clear from these examples that there is no one 'hierarchy of evidence' that works for all research questions. Therefore you should treat any claim that there is just 'one hierarchy of evidence' with some discernment. As suggested above, it is far better if you identify your 'own hierarchy of evidence' (Aveyard 2010), according to what evidence you need to address your own situation or problem.

What about using secondary sources?

Secondary sources are those that report the findings of other people's work without giving full details of the work they discuss.

A secondary source is a source that does not report the data from a primary research study directly but it might refer to the study without giving full details. A secondary source is therefore a step removed from the ideas you are referring to.

For example: a report in the *British Medical Journal* (BMJ) might refer to a systematic review published by the Cochrane Collaboration. The BMJ report would be the secondary source and the Cochrane Collaboration report the primary source. You may see it written as: Author A (2009) cited in Author B (2010)

- You are advised to access the primary source wherever possible and the use of **secondary sources should be avoided** wherever possible.
- If you rely on a secondary report and you do not access the original report, there is potential for you to miss any error in the way in which the initial source was reported and interpreted.
- Therefore where you need to quote from another source, you are always advised to **access the original** paper rather than to refer to a report of it, unless it is not possible to get hold of the primary source, for example if it is out of print or an unpublished doctoral thesis.

Let's say that the author (Author B) of a paper you are reading cites the work of a well-known author (Author A) who has done a lot of work in the area. If you refer to the work of Author A without accessing the original work, you are using a secondary source. You are relying on the interpretation of Author B to inform you about the work of Author A. You can see that this could lead to a case of 'Chinese whispers' and this is why it should be avoided. Unless you read the original work by Author A directly, you are relying on Author B's interpretation of this work.

This means that you cannot comment on the way it is represented, the full context or upon the strengths and limitations of the original work.

Access this example of the pitfalls of using secondary sources without accessing the primary source (Bradshaw and Price 2006).

We will not describe their work here (that would make us a secondary source). So . . . we suggest you read it for yourselves.

Use of policy and guidelines

There are a range of guidelines and policies that you are likely to come across. Ideally, these guidelines and policies are developed from the best available evidence. They should be written in a user-friendly way so that you can apply the evidence easily in your professional setting.

There are some useful websites for **national guidance and policy** available at http://www.evidence.nhs.uk/ and there is a public health section too, available at http://www.evidence.nhs.uk/nhs-evidence-content/public-health

There is also a wide range of local, national and international guidance available for health and social care practitioners.

Evidence Updates highlight new evidence relating to published accredited guidance. They do not replace current guidance and do not provide formal practice recommendations. It is organized by topic: http://www.evidence.nhs.uk/nhs-evidence-content/evidence-updates

NHS Evidence also provides a link to **National Institute for Health and Clinical Excellence (NICE)** (http://www.evidence.nhs.uk/nhs-evidence-content/nice-and-nhs-evidence). NICE guidance claims to set the standards for high quality healthcare and to encourage healthy living. They state that their guidance 'can be used by the NHS, Local Authorities, employers, voluntary groups and anyone else involved in delivering care or promoting wellbeing'.

There are also **NICE quality standards** (http://www.nice.org.uk/aboutnice/qualitystandards/qualitystandards.jsp). NICE quality standards are said to be 'central to supporting the Government's vision for an NHS and Social Care system focussed on delivering the best possible outcomes for people who use services, as detailed in the Health and Social Care Act (2012)'. *http://www.legislation.gov.uk/ukpga/2012/7/enacted.* There are some quality standards for social work in development too.

NICE Pathways provides 'quick and easy access, topic by topic, to the range of guidance published by NICE, including quality standards, technology appraisals, clinical and public health guidance and NICE implementation tools'. They assert that pathways are simple to navigate and allow users to explore in increasing detail NICE recommendations and advice, giving the user confidence that they are up to date (http://pathways.nice.org.uk/).

Map of medicine health guides shows the ideal, evidence-based patient journey for common and important conditions. It claims to be a high-level overview to be used by professionals that can be shared with patients (http://healthguides.mapofmedicine.com/choices/map/index.html).

There are also clinical and professional guidelines specific to individual professions and sometimes specific disorders.

Check your own organization for evidence-based policy or guidelines. It is also worth accessing societies, colleges and organizations specific to your profession or specialty.

You might also find that research evidence is integrated into other user-friendly publications. This means that you do not always have to find the 'raw' data from the research but instead you find publications which have used the evidence that is relevant to a particular context. Examples of such publications are:

- Government or professional organizations' policy, reports, guidance or standards
- National Institute for Health and Clinical Excellence Guidelines which are compiled with close reference to Cochrane and Campbell Collaboration reviews
- Care pathways or protocols
- Results from audits
- Reports from international, national or local organizations
- Information from trusted websites
- Patient/client information leaflets.

As with other forms of evidence it is important that these forms of evidence are evaluated – this is explored further in Chapter 6.

Non-research-based evidence

As we have stated before, there will not always be evidence available for the area you seek. This may be in situations where you are unable to identify a focussed question you can 'ask of the literature'. This may be where there is complexity, circumstances or context that are individual to the particular patient/client or situation or where you really need to decide or act in a 'one off' situation. In this case, you may use alternate forms of evidence (such as intuition, expert opinion, reflective judgement or discussion papers and so on) to address the question you seek to answer at that moment. In this case, it is especially important that you assess the quality of the evidence that you have as we will discuss in Chapter 6. When you use non-research evidence in your assignments (if it is all that is available) or practice (because of time or complexity issues) be clear that you are aware that it is not strong evidence *even if it is the best available* and that you know about the limitations in the quality of evidence you are using. If you can you should at a later point find out if there is better quality direct or indirect research evidence that would better inform your practice next time.

In summary

There is a wide range of research evidence that you are likely to encounter when you seek evidence to answer questions that arise in your practice. It is important that you can recognize different types of research and understand when and why different approaches are used. There is no easy formula for determining what evidence is best in any given context – you need to consider carefully the types of evidence that will meet your needs. There is no one hierarchy of evidence; we suggest you develop your own for any given situation.

We will discuss how you search for and make sense of what you come across in the next two chapters. It is important that you are aware that different types of research evidence will assist you in addressing different types of questions that arise in practice.

Key points

1 You are likely to encounter a wide range of research and other information that is relevant to your specific question.
2 It is important that you can understand the key characteristics of a piece of research.
3 It is important to identify the types of research and other information that you need to address your question.
4 You may come across a wide range of evidence – what is important is that you can recognize what you read and use it appropriately.
5 Traditional hierarchies of evidence only apply if you are looking for evidence of effectiveness.
6 Try to consider what the hierarchy of evidence is for your particular situation or context.
7 Other forms of information besides research are available, but you should ensure they are of the highest quality and – *where they can b*e – are based on the best available evidence.

5

How do I find relevant evidence to support my practice and learning?

Focussing the topic area and refining the question • Using PICOT • Searching for relevant evidence • The importance of a comprehensive approach to searching for literature • How to develop an effective search strategy • In summary • Key points

In this chapter we will consider

- What evidence to look for – identifying your focus/keywords/search terms
- How to use the internet, databases and library
- How to search for literature
- How to increase, refine or reduce the results of a search
- How to use more advanced searching: hints and tips
- Using experts, specialists and colleagues
- What to include and what to reject.

Where do I find relevant information?

There are two things you need to do to find relevant information:

1. Focus the topic and refine the question
2. Search for evidence

In this chapter we will look at each of these things in turn.

Focussing the topic and refining the question

You may have a broad idea of the topic, relating to a decision you have made or need to make, but have yet to identify what exactly you need to focus on to answer your question. You may have a more specific interest in mind which has arisen from your academic studies, or an assignment you need to write, or an issue that has arisen in practice. We have already emphasized that the evidence you search for will depend on the question you need to answer. However it is also important to refine what you need to find out so that you are not inundated with information.

In Chapter 2 we discussed the information revolution and how as practitioners we are inundated with information about our practice. If you undertake searches on 'large' topics such as diabetes, child protection or depression you will get a very large number of results (hits) from your search and the results will seem unmanageable. You have probably found this already when undertaking search engine searches (such as Google). If you ask for information on a particular country or event, you may get thousands of hits. When you refine this to something more specific you probably come nearer to finding what you are looking for. It is the same within health and social care.

Consider what area of practice you are exploring. Your enquiry may relate to: assessment, screening, diagnosis, prognosis, prevention, interventions, management, outcomes, cost-benefits, patient/client/service user or staff or student experience, and so on. If you are searching for information, it helps to break down the topic into an aspect of the topic. For example, 'blood sugar level control in diabetes' or 'children's reaction to child protection services' or 'depression in the older person'.

It is important to be really clear about *what you want to find out* before you start looking in order to be more efficient with your time.

Refine the question

Once you have identified your topic area, you need to focus down further so that you have a specific area. Try and **put your enquiry into the form of a question** that you need to answer. This means that you seek an answer to a specific question rather than seeking information about the entire topic. There are many approaches you can take when you are **starting to define the question.** Sometimes what you need to search for is not immediately clear and it might help to think around the topic. You could:

- Think through/reflecting on your practice to isolate what really concerns you
- Talk to experts

- Brainstorm ideas with colleagues
- Use a spider diagram or mind map
- Carry out a quick initial database search
- Use a search engine to see broadly what terms/subjects come up. Google Scholar can be a good place to start http://scholar.google.co.uk/ as it is more specific and you can set filters by date etc.

Examples from practice:

Example 1: If you were searching for information regarding the attitudes of occupational therapists to dementia then you would need to select this professional group and also specify that you were exploring attitudes, not the effectiveness of interventions.

Example 2: If you were looking for evidence about the outcomes for children at risk who were moved out of the family home, then you would need to look specifically at these children rather than children at risk who were not removed from the home.

Example 3: If you are wondering why your patient/client's leg ulcer is not responding to the treatment you are giving and you have heard that using Manuka honey might be effective in the healing process, you therefore might want to look specifically at the effectiveness of Manuka honey.

In addition to focussing down on a specific question, it is also useful to consider exactly what type of evidence will help you address your question. In Chapter 3 we discussed how different problems need different types of evidence and you need to be clear about what you are looking for.

Example 4: If you want to know whether or not an intervention or programme works, then you need to look for RCTs or reviews of these studies in the first instance.

Example 5: If you want to know how about a patient or client's experience with a particular condition or situation, then you could look for phenomenological studies or reviews of these studies in the first instance.

Focussing and structuring your question using PICOT (or PICO)

Consider using the acronym **PICOT** when you are identifying the question you want to address. Do note that the sections of PICOT have different meanings depending on whether you are looking for quantitative or qualitative research. Also you may come across the acronym PICO which has the same meaning but has the last stage omitted. Fineout-Overholt and Johnston (2005) and Stillwell *et al.* (2010) suggest the two following stages of defining a question, depending on the type of research we are looking for:

Standard PICOT	Qualitative PICOT
Population	Population
Intervention	Issue
Comparison	Context
Outcome	Outcome
Time	Time

These can be explained as follows:

Population: We need to consider who are the people we are interested in investigating with similar characteristics such as gender, age, condition, problem, location and role. For example, older people in residential care, those who are homeless, mothers under 45, patients/clients who have had knee replacements, patient/clients who have accessed paramedic services for chest pain, staff who work out of hours, students who access study advice.

Intervention/issue (quantitative/qualitative): These can be diagnostic, therapeutic, preventative, exposure, managerial, experiences, perceptions, costs and so on.

Comparisons/context (quantitative/qualitative): This can be against another intervention or no intervention; comparisons can be made against national or professional standards or guidelines. The context of the study can be where the study takes place or factors that impact on an experience.

Outcome: Faster, cheaper, reasons why, reduction or increase in, for example: symptoms, benefits, events, episodes, prognosis, mortality, accuracy. For qualitative studies outcome may be the experiences or attitudes.

Time: This may or may not be relevant, for example: three days postoperative or five hours post-intervention, within 24 hours of accessing the service.

Example of PICOT question (quantitative): Does education about smoking *(intervention)* **reduce smoking** *(outcome)* **in young people** *(population)* **in state education** *(comparison if there is a control group of those who did not receive education)* **before the age of 16** *(time)*?

> **Example of PICOT question (qualitative): Why** *(outcome)* **do young people** *(population)* **in state education** *(context)* **start smoking** *(issue)* **before the age of 16** *(time)?*

Try writing a research question using the PICOT process on something you want to explore in your practice.

Once you have identified what you are trying to find out, you need to consider what evidence will enable you to answer the question. Whilst appreciating which research approaches are most likely to be relevant to answering your research question, you are advised to remain open minded at this stage about the inclusion of all types of information if they are relevant to your research question.

Searching for relevant evidence

Once you have established the specific topic or question you want to answer (*research question*) you need to develop an effective approach to your search (*search strategy*) that will enable you to identify and locate the widest range and most relevant publications within your time and financial limitations.

The importance of a comprehensive approach to searching for literature

If you are comprehensive or systematic in your approach to searching for literature, you are likely to access the best available evidence. If you do not adopt a systematic approach, you are likely to access a random selection of literature.

What's wrong with Google? Internet search engines such as Google are **not** specific enough to search effectively although they may give you some ideas of language terms used. This is why you need to access a **subject specific search engine or database**.

- A literature search that is approached systematically is very different from one that is approached in a haphazard manner!
- A thorough and comprehensive search strategy will help to ensure that you identify all the key literature/texts and research on your topic.
- If you are using the information to share with others or in your writing then documenting your stated strategy will ensure that those who access your evidence know what you looked for, what was included and excluded and where you searched.

Think about how you might have accessed literature in the past for your learning and for your practice and consider the pros and cons of these approaches.

You may have found literature in your workplace from a search engine or website or obtained it from colleagues. Or you might have carried out a quick search and used the first thing you found. Some examples of information sources that are 'easy to access' but which may not give you a comprehensive account of evidence in the area are:

- Newspapers and other forms of media
- Websites focussing on health and social care
- Internet search engines such as Google and Yahoo!
- Lectures and lecture notes
- Lecturers or practice assessor/mentors
- Colleagues in your professional practice area
- Journals to which your workplace/learning institution has a subscription.

Although in fast-paced situations with little time you may draw on some of these sources, where a situation or issue is likely to reoccur, it is better to undertake a more thorough search.

Potential problems with haphazard/casual approaches to finding literature

- It could be out of date.
- It could be biased.
- You may miss out on finding key literature.
- It may not be the best available evidence for the question you have.
- Contradictory literature may be out there.
- It may present only one part of the whole picture.
- Harder-to-find literature may be really useful in answering your question.
- Your conclusions are likely to be inaccurate.

In another publication (Aveyard *et al.* 2011) we discuss the difference between information that is readily available and information that is the best available.

You can see here the limitations of relying on haphazard or casual approaches to finding and using evidence – you will not find a comprehensive or full range of evidence on the topic you are interested in, however useful it is to get ideas from journals that you come across in the office, department etc. There is likely to be far more evidence available and what you have may be 'just the tip if the iceberg'.

How to develop an effective search strategy

We suggest the following steps in developing a **search strategy:**

1 Be clear about the research question or problem you need to address.
2 Identify your key terms and inclusion and exclusion criteria.
3 Define the inclusion and exclusion criteria.
4 Undertake a comprehensive search using your key terms and inclusion and exclusion criteria.
5 Record your search strategy.
6 Manage and store your literature effectively.

We now look at each step in turn.

1. Be clear about the focus of your literature search

If you articulate your focus at the beginning of the searching process, this will help to keep you on track. State your enquiry as a question as this will help you to stay focussed. It is important to ensure that you only find that information which is relevant to the research question and it is very easy to get sidetracked, so it is useful to use the PICOT or PICO formula as described above to form a clear question.

2. Identify your key terms/keywords

Once you have articulated the focus of your literature search, you need to identify some key terms for which you can search for literature. You will use these key terms when you come to search using the databases, and identifying the terms in the first instance will help you clarify the purpose of your search. The databases you use retrieve information by **keywords** and it is important to identify these in advance. You need to think laterally when you do this – try to think of the different ways in which your topic could be referred to and identify the keywords that you think are likely to represent your topic. Google can help you to do this, as you will see the different ways that your topic is discussed and the phrases that are used. You can also use the **thesaurus** component, **subject index** or **MeSH** terms or **topic tree** of a database search engine. These help you to identify more keywords that you may not have thought of initially. You can also refer to other published literature in the area to find out how the authors of other papers have searched using keywords. You will find that your search for evidence is not a one-off process but an evolving process that you return to and refine as your ideas develop.

- You should be as creative as possible as the topic or question might be categorized in different ways by different researchers.
- Think of all the words that may mean the same thing (use a thesaurus if you can, they are often accessible on the database itself).
- Consider different spellings of the same word (US and UK) and/or if the endings may vary i.e. children/child/children's (see below).
- You also need to consider whether there are different meanings in different countries of the keywords that you identify, especially given that databases have different biases. For example, CINAHL has a strong North American bias and the BNI has a British focus.
- Don't limit your keywords to terms that are conventional if you think literature might be indexed using different headings.
- You will find that you identify new possible search terms as your searching progresses.

For example: Consider the way in which the term 'learning difficulties/ disabilities' is used. Some people have strong feelings about which term is used. However, if you are searching for literature in this area, be careful to use every term that might have been used to index the literature or you risk omitting vital literature from your search.

---

3. Define your inclusion and exclusion criteria

Inclusion and exclusion criteria enable you to identify the literature that addresses the research question and to reject that which does not.

Once you have identified your key terms, you need to identify inclusion and exclusion criteria that will assist you in selecting appropriate literature for your topic. Whilst inclusion and exclusion criteria are generally used by those undertaking a search as part of a larger more formal literature review, the principles of including and excluding relevant/irrelevant literature apply to every literature search. The criteria you develop will be guided by the wording of your research question and your focus. Unless your question clearly indicates otherwise, you are likely to be looking for primary research or literature reviews in the first instance. You should be able to justify why you have set the inclusion and exclusion criteria, which should be determined by the needs of the question you need to answer rather than your own convenience. For example, it would not be appropriate to include only studies which are available electronically if a hard paper copy of an article you require is available in the local library.

Example of inclusion criteria:

- Primary research directly related to the topic
- English language only
- Published literature only
- 2008 onwards
- In a particular setting or a particular population

Example of exclusion criteria:

- Primary research not directly related to the topic area
- Non-English language
- Unpublished research
- Pre- 2008
- Not in a particular setting or with a particular population

Should I limit my search for practical reasons?

In an ideal world, you would be able to search and locate all the information that is relevant to your specific topic and/or the question you are addressing. However, some of your criteria will be set for practical reasons, such as time and resources.

> **Example:** Practicalities might mean you have to limit your search to recent literature and omit unpublished literature from your search. Neither of these restrictions are ideal and you might lose relevant literature – there might be a piece of work which is highly relevant to your review but which was published before the date limitations you set.

If you set time restrictions to your search for literature you would miss this key document, although it might be referred to in other papers. You should not limit a search to only access electronic **full text availability**, as even if you find it difficult to physically visit your library, most libraries will offer a photocopying service.

Should I limit my search to published literature only?

Again, in an ideal world, you would seek to access all available literature on your topic or research question. There might be a lot of 'hidden' evidence about your topic that remains unpublished, called **'grey literature'**. Non-academic journals might also be referred to as grey literature and other information such as policies also falls into this category.

Remember that exclusion criteria will reduce the number of results (hits) you get whereas inclusion criteria will increase them.

4. Undertaking a comprehensive search

Once you have identified your question, keywords and inclusion and exclusion criteria, you are ready to begin searching for literature/evidence.

There are five main ways of searching for literature. These are:

- Electronic searching using computer-held databases
- Searching reference lists of articles you already have
- Hand searching relevant journals specific to the research topic or using electronic journal searching
- Contacting authors directly
- Searching national guidelines/professional body sites.

Computer held databases

Searching for literature has become a far easier and efficient process with the advent of electronic databases for literature searching. If you have recently visited your local academic or professional library, you will be very aware that the computer revolution has had a large impact on the ways in which we search for information. In the past (when we were students) those reviewing the literature would have to search through hard-bound volumes of subject indexed references in which previously published literature was categorized under various keywords. They could not be immediately updated and updates took place often on a yearly basis. Those seeking information had no alternative other than to trawl through bound volumes to find information on a topic or by an author (and then commonly, anything published within the last year was unobtainable because it was in the process of binding). Nowadays, most of the information you need is accessible through one of many databases.

What are databases?

In general there are two types of database often referred to in the literature searching process.

Subject specific databases (e.g. MEDLINE) contain references for your topic of interest and allow you to search for that information, normally in the form of published academic papers (journal articles). These databases are compiled as follows: published papers are scrutinized and allocated keywords which are then indexed. This index of keywords is then stored by the database. When you come to search the database, you enter a keyword and the database produces a list of references of the papers it holds which have been allocated your keyword. Normally, the reference is given in the form of name, date of publication, title of publication, title of journal in which the information is held and possibly an abstract for the paper. As an added bonus, some databases provide a link to an electronic copy of the full version of the paper. If not you can use the electronic journal databases described below.

Electronic journal databases are useful when you know exactly what you are looking for and have a reference for a particular journal article. You can locate the journal you need and from that you can locate the particular article you need to get hold of. It is usually organized via an A–Z section which contains access to the electronic copy of the papers (journal articles). It is important to note that the electronic journal database does not allow you to search for what is written on your topic (the subject specific database is better for this) but is useful to locate the sources identified from the subject specific databases.

Getting started using databases

Identify relevant databases to which you have access. Various health and social care databases will be available through professional websites, university or organizational libraries to which you belong. Different databases access literature from different countries or groups of countries or focus on specific specialities or interest areas. You need to ensure you use an appropriate one.

- Find out if you need a password to access these and set one up. Your librarian will help with this.
- Familiarize yourself with the way in which each database works and do note that all databases operate differently – do not assume that commands you use for one database will be understood by another.
- Access any help sheets or online tutorials or go for a training session on searching.

Cochrane have a collection of databases in their **'webliography'** available at http://www.cochrane.org/about-us/evidence-based-health-care/webliography/databases

---

Commonly held specific databases include:

AMED: allied health including occupational therapy, physiotherapy, complementary therapy, and palliative care.

ASSIA: Applied Social Sciences Indexes and Abstracts.

Autism Data: open access database of over 18,500 published research papers, books, articles and videos on Autism.

British Nursing Index: information about nursing, midwifery and community healthcare, mainly from UK journals.

CAB Abstracts: human nutrition, biotechnology, infectious diseases.

Campbell Collaboration: systematic reviews of the effects of social interventions, such as education, crime and justice and social welfare. It is an American database, freely available on and off campus.

Cancer Library: compiled by the National Cancer Institute in the USA.

CASonline: provided by the British Institute of Learning Disabilities. To connect you will need a password.

CINAHL: nursing and allied healthcare from North America and Europe.

CIRRIE: Centre for International Rehabilitation Research Information and Exchange database.

Cochrane Library: evidence-based healthcare (systematic reviews of evidence for the effectiveness of treatments).

DARE (Database of Abstracts of Reviews of Effects): abstracts of systematic reviews covering effects of interventions. You need to tick the box to restrict your search to DARE.

DUETs: Database of Uncertanties about the Effects of Treatments.

HMIC: non-clinical topics including inequalities in health and user involvement, health services and hospital administration, management and policy.

Joanna Briggs Institute: systematic reviews, evidence summaries and best practice information sheets in nursing and allied health from the Joanna Briggs Institute.

MEDLINE: connect via Ebsco, PubMed or Web of Knowledge. Extensive medical and nursing database.

OpenSigle: open access to SIGLE bibliographical references of reports and other grey literature produced in Europe until 2005.

OTdirect: study notes, practice updates and training listings produced by OTs in their spare time.

OTseeker: abstracts of systematic reviews and Randomized Controlled Trials relevant to occupational therapy.

PEDRO: physiotherapy evidence database.

Planex: Local public policy and governance including social work. Covers material published since 1980.

PsychINFO: psychology, psychiatry, child development, psychological aspects of illness and treatment.

PubMed: extensive medical, biomedical and nursing database. Freely available on and off campus.

NARIC (National Rehabilitation Information Center): disability and rehabilitation databases.

National Research Register Archive: a database of research projects funded by, or of interest to the NHS, collected until September 2007.

NHS Clinical Knowledge Summaries: evidence based information on common conditions managed in primary care.

Rehabdata: disability and rehabilitation produced by the (US) National Rehabilitation Information Center.

Social Care Online: social and community care, includes Department of Health circulars.

Social Services Abstracts: abstracts from journal articles on social work, welfare and policy.

Sociological Abstracts: sociology and political theory.

Source: management and practice of primary healthcare and disability in developing countries.

TRIP database: evidence-based medicine and healthcare resources on the web.

Web of Science: includes Science Citation Index and Social Sciences Citation Index.

ZETOC: British Library's electronic table of contents. Covers about 20,000 current journals and conference proceedings in many key subject areas.

(This is just a selection; your own library may have others.)

You may find it useful to use a table such as the one below which helps identify and structure your search from your PICOT question.

The general technique is as follows:

Use Boolian operators. Make sure you make use of the **AND/OR** commands in the searching strategy as appropriate. The use of AND, OR and NOT are called **Boolean operators.**

AND ensures that **each** term you have entered is searched for. This will reduce the number of hits you get as each term must be included in the article for it to be recognized.

OR ensures that **either one term or another** is selected. This will increase the number of hits you get as you only need to identify one of the terms for the article to be selected.

If you keep getting results that are not useful you may wish to use **NOT** to **exclude** specific topics.

There is also the '*** facility**' which enables you to identify all possible endings of the key term you write. You need to identify the 'root' of the word for example, the part of the word that doesn't change – and put the * after that last letter. For example: child* will identify articles containing child, children, children's and so on. The **Wildcard** replaces one or more letters in a word. For example, for woman or women the wildcard is 'Wom?n'.

Remember that it takes time to get to accustomed to database searching. If you are a practice assessor/mentor, ask your student to show you how to search.

Example question: What is the **attitude** of **student** (nurse or other **profession**) to **HIV/AIDS?**

	1 Keyword		2 Keyword		3 Keyword		4 Keyword
a)	Attitude*	AND	Student*	AND	Nurse (or state other profession)	AND	Human immunodeficiency virus
	Or		Or		Or		Or
b)	Stigma		Baccalaureate*		Nurs*		HIV
	Or		Or				Or
c)	Approach*		Undergraduate*				H.I.V.
	Or		Or				or
d)	Opinion*		Pre-registration				Acquired immunodeficiency syndrome
	Or		Or				or
e)	View*		Pre-qualifying				AIDS

Adapted from Oldershaw (2009)

Try and identify search terms for a question you have using this table (you can add rows or columns as you need to). Column 5 may be used to record the number of hits (or results).

1 Keyword		2 Keyword		3 Keyword		4 Keyword	5 No. of hits
Or	AND	or	AND	or	AND	or	
Or		or		or		or	
Or		or		or		or	

You can specify whether you would like to search throughout *the whole article* for the term, or whether you are going to limit your search to the *abstract* (the short summary) or just the *title*.

- If you limit your search to the identification of the term in just the title, you will exclude a lot of references which might be relevant to you, as some titles will not use the key terms you have identified.
- If you search through the whole articles for your keyword, you are likely to be overwhelmed with literature.
- Limiting your search to the abstract is likely to be a suitable compromise.
- If you get few articles on a less common or unusual keyword you may want to search in the whole article.

You are likely to need to refine your searching strategy as you progress. You will find that you will develop new ideas as you undertake the searching process. You might find, for example, a key theme is called by a different name or phrase that you had not previously thought of. Be aware of this and be prepared to search using new and different terms.

Once you have identified the key literature on your topic using one database, you could repeat the search using another database. This will depend on the requirements of your search. If you find that the same references are thrown up, then you can be confident that your strategy is well focussed and that you are accessing the relevant literature on your topic. You might feel it is appropriate to scale down your search.

Getting help

Your subject librarian at your university or hospital will be happy to guide you. In this chapter we discuss database searching and your local library is likely to provide tutorials or help sheets in searching for evidence. When you get started you will find academic journals relating to a very wide range of professional interests. Some journals are generic to the interests of one professional group – for example *Journal of Clinical Nursing* or *British Journal of Occupational Therapy*, whilst others are specialist journals belonging to a particular area of professional interest for example *Addiction*. Academic journals contain many articles about different topics related to the overall subject addressed by the journal.

There are now an increasing number of **specialist evidence-based practice journals** such as: *World Views on Evidence-based Nursing, Evidence-based Mental Health, Journal of Evidence-based Dental Health, Evidenced-based Complementary and Alternative Medicine, Journal of Evidence-based Social Work, Evidence-based Child Health, International Journal of Evidence-based Health Care, Evidence-based Midwifery.*

Journals often contain a mixture of research, literature reviews and discussion/ opinion articles, which we will discuss later on in this book in more depth.

Remember . . .

- Searching for literature is time consuming and needs skill – you are advised not to leave it until the last minute before searching.
- If you do not have any 'hits' from your search, then you need to keep searching with different keywords until you identify literature which is linked to your topic area. If you have too many hits, you will need to refocus your search.
- Remember to keep a record of the search terms you have used and the results of these searches.

If new references are constantly being thrown up, you will need to continue searching until later searches reveal little or no new information.

Why is electronic searching not 100 per cent effective?

Despite the advances in electronic searching, computerized searching tools are not 100 per cent effective and will fail to identify some of the relevant literature on your topic.

This is because:

- Some relevant literature might have been categorized using different keywords and would therefore not be identified by one particular search strategy.
- The topic you are looking for may be mentioned in several papers but not to a large extent and therefore was not indexed when these papers were entered on to the database. This means that the papers will not be recognized by the databases when you search for this topic.
- You may have only searched within the title of articles.
- The title may be misleading.

Authors who use imaginative titles for their work run the risk that their work will not be identified by those who search on the topic. Although using various keywords will help identify literature that is not identified on the first search, it is still possible for literature to remain unidentified even though it is highly relevant to addressing the research question.

Is searching for evidence an art or a science?

We have emphasized that searching for evidence will never be a one-off process. You will need to ensure you have strived for a thorough coverage of the available evidence and continue to update and refine your searches. The more you search, the more you will begin to develop instinct and experience about where to search and what terms are used around your subject matter. **Knowledge of your subject matter** will certainly help with this.

> **Example:** an inexperienced searcher may search for 'use of gloves AND aprons' in infection control. A more experienced individual will recognize that it may be better to search under the terms 'universal OR standard precautions' rather than seek out the individual protective equipment.

Therefore, you should regard searching for evidence as both a science and an art. Searching should be regarded as a science, because we encourage you to undertake a **methodological and comprehensive** approach to the identification of relevant evidence. Searching should also be regarded as an art because you also need to be **creative and flexible** about the way you identify relevant evidence.

Searching the reference lists

Once you have identified the key articles that relate to your research question, you might want to scrutinize the reference lists of those **key articles** for further references that may be useful to you. You will use the same keywords and inclusion and exclusion criteria to do this, although you may come across important older key texts, which are frequently referenced, but that fall outside your exclusion dates.

Hand-searching relevant journals

If you have been able to identify that many of your key articles which are relevant to your research question are located in one or two journals, it might be useful to hand-search these journals to see whether you can identify other relevant articles that have not been identified through other searching strategies. Searching through the contents pages of these journals may identify other relevant material. This may also be done electronically through an A–Z of journals and selecting the relevant journal (some journal websites have archive search facilities).

Author searching/using experts

If you find that many of your key articles are by the same author(s) then it may be useful to carry out an author search in order to identify whether the author(s) have published other work which has not been identified in the electronic search. This might also lead you towards work in progress. In some specialist areas it may be worth contacting the author directly to see if they are aware of any other sources. **Experts** in a clinical or professional area may have attended conferences or be involved in projects that address your issue or question. Contacting them directly may highlight new sources. If they have been helpful, it is considered polite to share your findings with them once your research is complete. If your topic includes a product or service then the manufacturers/suppliers may have commissioned research. You need to be aware of the potential bias of such research.

Grey literature

Grey literature is a term used to describe literature that has not been published and is therefore hard to find. If the area is under researched, you might find that useful grey literature does exist. You can identify this literature in a number of ways, such as contacting known authors in an area and asking if they know of other sources of information. However, use of grey literature is unlikely to be a main component of your literature search.

Professional body or government publications

Remember that your professional body will have many resources and it will be useful to look at these to find additional sources of information. In health and social care there may be government policy or legislation that can provide a useful addition to your search strategy.

A **combination of these searching strategies** will ensure that you have the most comprehensive search strategy and therefore the most chance of retrieving the information that is relevant to your research question. However, you can never be certain that you have obtained all the literature on a particular topic. Greenhalgh and Peacock (2005) refer to this process as **'snowball sampling'** where you are pointed in the direction of additional literature from your existing literature. For example, if useful articles are found in a particular journal, then this journal is further scrutinized for other relevant material. This strategy cannot be pre-specified and is dependent on the results of early literature searching.

How to use abstracts to confirm the relevance of the paper

Once you have identified the literature that is relevant to you, the next step is to sort through the reference list you now have and identify which references are most relevant. To do this, you **cannot rely on the title** alone. This is because the focus of the article, whether or not it is a primary research study, is often unclear from the title alone.

 The *abstract* will give you a summary of the content of the article, in particular whether it is a research article or not.

The abstract is often available on the electronic databases such as CINAHL or MEDLINE. However, abstracts can themselves be unreliable sources for determining the exact focus of a paper, and you might find that you miss relevant literature if you discard a paper because of the information contained in the abstract. However, given that you are unlikely to be able to access in full each paper you identify from an electronic search, you will have to rely on the abstract to determine whether or not the paper will address your research question. If you cannot tell from the abstract, you will need to access the paper in order to do this.

Getting hold of your sources from the references

The references to which you are directed are likely to be found in journals, books and other publications.

You can **find journal articles** in a variety of ways:

- Accessing the journal archives via their website or sometimes a search engine on the internet
- Accessing an electronic library using the internet, with a password supplied by your librarian
- Accessing the paper copies (often referred to as hard copies) in your library.

 Try to get training on using your local library (especially from a subject specialist) to help you locate publications.

- Most university and workplace libraries will have many journals accessible as **'full-text'** electronically and you will find that you can locate and download many articles without leaving your computer. **You will need a password to access these.** There is sometimes – but not always – a link from the database to the full text article in the electronic library.
- You are strongly advised to familiarize yourself with the journals to which you have easy access through your local library. Some libraries will have a subject specific catalogue.
- If the reference you require is not available full-text electronically, then you will need to access the bound volumes which are available as hard copies in the library.
- If the references are not available electronically or in bound volumes in your local library, then you will need to either arrange to visit another library or arrange an **inter-library loan.** This will have a small cost and be time consuming so you will need to make a decision about the effort you go to.
- It may be worth trying a general internet search for the article as increasingly articles are posted on websites. Do make sure it is the complete original article (best as a pdf file) and that it has not been summarized or altered.

Strengths and limitations of your searching strategy

Clearly, those doing a more detailed systematic review need to make every effort to retrieve the articles relevant to their study. Those undertaking a smaller scale literature search do not need to go to the same lengths to retrieve literature, although of course the more comprehensive the search, the better. Overall, your search will be more comprehensive the more effort you make in locating all the references that are central to your question.

Some potential limitations of a search:

Experience of the researchers. If you are doing a project by yourself, you are unlikely to have the same skills and resources as a team of people working together. Those working together can share ideas, read abstracts and papers together and so on. If you are a novice researcher you are more likely to miss sources than a more experienced researcher.

Potential bias. You should identify any potential bias of the sources you used – if you have been unable to track down certain sources, you should acknowledge this. If you have limited your sources by accessibility then this is a limitation, or if papers you find are sponsored by companies or organizations that may influence the results, this should be recognized.

5. Recording your searching strategy

It may be helpful to keep a record of your searching strategy, the keywords or combinations of words that you used and the number of hits, so that you can demonstrate a systematic approach.

See the table on page 100 and consider using one of the columns to record the number of hits. This may be of particular use for academic assignments or if you are sharing the results of your search with other professionals/colleagues as evidence for your practice. The reader should clearly be able to see how you refined your search and got to the final ones that you reviewed. A systematic search should be able to be repeated by someone else who would find the exact same papers.

Example: If you are searching for primary research articles concerned with smoking and social care, you might initially undertake two basic searches and then combine these searches:

Databases: CINAHL 1994 – Search term: smok*: Total number of hits: 30,000

Databases: CINAHL 1994 – Search term: smok* AND social care* Total number of hits: 15,000

You can then demonstrate how you combined this search with another search in order to obtain a more manageable number of hits.

It might also be useful to demonstrate the success of your searching strategy and which searches yielded the best results. It is also useful to state what type of literature your hits included, if you can determine this from the abstract available. If you are searching for articles of primary research but are failing to identify these, you can document this.

Tips for documenting your search strategy

- Remember that the aim is to demonstrate how you undertook a **systematic approach** to your searching.
- Discuss **the approach** you took to develop an effective search strategy.
- **Keep a record** of all the search terms used so that you can provide evidence of your approach if asked.
- Keep a record of the **other approaches** you employed to search for literature.
- Be able to comment on the **effectiveness** of the approaches you used. For example, if electronic searching did not yield as many hits as you had hoped, discuss why this might have been.
- Make every effort to **obtain** relevant literature.
- It is more accurate to write '*I did not find any literature on X*' rather than categorically '*there is no literature . . .*'

It is recommended that you avoid statements in your writing that declare that there is no literature on a particular topic and state instead, if asked, that *no literature was identified* on the topic in question.

Remember to:

- Back up (save) all your records and keep them in a safe place throughout your searching process.
- Keep records on more than one site (what if your computer was stolen or there was a fire?) and consider emailing a copy of your reference list to yourself.
- If you are using full text electronic copies of articles then set up a folder so they are all together.
- Write references down in full every time you read something useful. It is very frustrating to have to track down page numbers or editions of references you have mislaid.
- Some people choose to keep a card filing system for all references.
- Consider using a reference manager such as ENDNOTE which will hold all your references electronically and produce a reference list in the format you require.
- A clear record should show how you got to the articles you are using to underpin your conclusions and so it could be repeated by someone else who would identify the same articles.

> You need to determine if you have found sufficient, appropriate evidence to answer your question.

A single source of evidence that has not been 'judged' or appraised for its quality is generally not enough. We will consider this aspect of evidence further as we go through this book.

In summary

You should by now be well aware of the importance of a systematic search strategy. This will ensure that you access a comprehensive range of literature that is relevant to your question. The use of inclusion and exclusion criteria can be very useful in ensuring that the literature identified is relevant to your review question. The need to combine the electronic searching of relevant databases with additional strategies such as hand-searching journals and examining reference lists has been discussed. You need to be aware that electronic searching can never be fully comprehensive and that 'snowball sampling', using many different strategies to identify literature will usually be the most effective way of achieving the most comprehensive literature search. At the end of the searching process, you will achieve a list of references that are relevant to your research question which you will be able to locate in your academic/professional library.

At this point, you should be confident that you have identified the most relevant literature that will enable you to answer your research question. You should be aware of the strengths and limitations of your search strategy and be prepared to justify your approach if asked. It is now time to stand back and take a critical look at the literature you have identified. We will discuss how you can do this in the next chapter.

Key points

1 You need a focussed question in order to identify your search terms.
2 It is important to identify the types of literature that will enable you to answer your research question.
3 Inclusion and exclusion criteria should be specific to your question.
4 The literature search strategy should incorporate a variety of approaches including electronic searching, hand-searching and reference list searching.
5 The limitations of these approaches should be acknowledged.

6

How do I know if the evidence is convincing and useful?

What is critical appraisal? • The importance of critical appraisal • Defining the terms used in judging quality • Getting started with critical appraisal • Getting to know your literature • General critical appraisal tools • Specific appraisal tools • Key questions for reviewing evidence • Key questions to ask of review articles • Key questions to ask of quantitative studies • Key questions to ask of qualitative studies • Key questions to ask of professional guidelines • Key questions to ask of discussion/opinion papers • Key questions to ask of websites • Incorporating critical appraisal into your academic writing and in practice • In summary • Key points

In the previous chapters, we have discussed how you identify the type of evidence that you need and how you find it. In this chapter, we will discuss how you know that you have found relevant information and how to recognize different types of evidence. We will also explore how you can tell if the information and evidence you find is 'any good' or not.

Overall we want you to move from a position where you would be tempted to say '*I've read this so it must be true*' to a position where you say '*I've read this – now I need to know if it is reliable*'. Specifically we will explore:

- Definitions of critical appraisal, its importance and key terms
- How to organize and identify the type of evidence you find from your literature search

- How to judge the quality and quantity of different sources of evidence we use (critical appraisal).

What is critical appraisal?

Critical appraisal is the structured process of examining a piece of evidence in order to *determine its strengths and limitations* and therefore the *relevance or weight* it should have in addressing your research question.

In a recent Cochrane review, Horsley *et al.* (2011: 4) draw on an early definition of critical appraisal by Last (1988):

> The process of assessing and interpreting evidence (usually published research) by systematically considering its validity (closeness to the truth), results and relevance to the individual's work.

In the review's 'plain language' summary they state that *'Critical appraisal involves interpreting information, in particular information within research papers, in a systematic and objective manner'* (Horsley *et al.* 2011: 1).

The common theme from these two definitions is that the appraiser needs to **interpret** what is read, i.e. not just accept it. This is vitally important, given the vast amount of information there is on any one topic and it illustrates the need to be both **selective and critical** of what you read. Any piece of evidence will not do – you need to make sure you are using the **best available** evidence.

When you critically appraise, you **evaluate or judge the quality and usefulness** of the evidence you have. This is the case whether you are writing an essay, a dissertation or using evidence directly in practice. The evidence you use will affect the quality of your academic work or the care provided in the clinical/professional environment.

There is a useful **overview guide to critical appraisal** in the 'what is' series (Burls 2009) (www.whatisseries.co.uk/whatis/pdfs/what_is_crit_appr.pdf).

Individual organizations such as **professional bodies or universities** sometimes offer explanations and guidance. For physiotherapists (although useful to all professions): http://www.csp.org.uk/professional-union/library/bibliographic-databases/critical-appraisal

For public health: http://www.healthknowledge.org.uk/public-health-textbook/frameworks/ca

---

The importance of critical appraisal

The controversy surrounding the measles, mumps and rubella (MMR) vaccination described in Chapter 4 illustrates the importance of undertaking critical appraisal of all research and other information that you encounter. The original publication that sparked the controversy was published in 1998 and the media scare is well known. It is difficult to find a better example of the need to be critical of published evidence. And in this case the evidence was published in a top ranking journal. Any practitioner who had read Wakefield's original article could see at a glance that the evidence it provided was not strong evidence – the research was carried out on 12 children and the circumstances in which the research was undertaken has caused several of the authors to retract their involvement in the study.

However none of this prevented the **media scare** that took over and there was evidence that practitioners become reluctant to administer the MMR vaccination and parents became reluctant to take their children for vaccination. The MMR controversy illustrates the **importance of critical appraisal** of research and other information so that you can identify how strong and relevant the evidence is relating to a particular topic.

Defining the terms used in judging the quality of research

When you are reading about critical appraisal, you will find many terms that come up time and time again. It is important to know what these mean. Their use can vary with the type of research.

You may find that the authors of the studies you read define any of these terms or include a glossary. It is important to know what we mean by these phrases, so here is a re-cap of the key terms:

- **Bias** – an error in the design or conduct of research which leads to the wrong result. For example, in an RCT you are comparing one treatment or intervention against another. If another aspect of care or treatment differs between the two arms of the trial and that changes the outcomes, this would be bias. This is why we try to use blinding in a trial so that this does not happen.
- **Credibility** – evidence that the results or conclusions are believable.
- **Generalizabilty** – findings of the research that can be applied to other people in other settings.
- **Relevance** – research that can be applied to any patient or client group and context.

- **Reliability** – the same results/conclusions would be found if the research was repeated.
- **Reproducibility** – the study or parts of the study could be repeated in other settings by other people.
- **Rigour** – evidence that the research has been carried out in a robust manner.
- **Transferability** – the results of a study may be transferred to another context or population.
- **Trustworthiness** – honest and reliable reporting of a study.
- **Validity** – the research accurately measures and reports what it says it does.

In addition:

- **Strengths** – refer to the good things about the literature, in relation to the points above.
- **Limitations** – refer to what could be criticized about the literature, in relation to the points above.

It is considered good practice for authors to identify some of the strengths and limitations themselves.

Getting started with critical appraisal

Every time you read the newspapers you probably form a judgement of whether or not you believe what you read; you might even wonder which sources were used to write the article. If you don't believe what you read, you might be tempted to track down the source upon which the article is based. Then what usually happens (well, for us anyway) is that you don't have time to research this further and you never really find out if what you read is true or not . . . Now consider the way you approach your professional reading. Just as we are sceptical about what we read in the papers, so we should be about what we read in the academic journals. This is the starting point of **critical appraisal.**

We should also think the same way about what we hear from colleagues or practice assessors/mentors. This will be discussed more in the next chapter.

 Refer back to how you have used literature or other forms of evidence in the past and consider the potential problems with your approach. Did you:

- Scan read it?
- Use only one or two sources?

- Only use what agreed with the point you wanted to make?
- Only use readily available sources?
- Copy literature without really understanding it?
- Ignore research that didn't agree with your current practice?
- Just use quotes or sections that agreed with your view?
- Believe everything that is written without questioning the authority of the writer or the quality of the arguments or evidence?

It is important not to fall into either of the following two categories:

1 **You accept any piece of research** or other information at face value and accept what is written without question. You may believe that a paper published in a high quality journal or written by an expert is above critique and so do not attempt any structured appraisal of the paper. Even a paper that is published in a reputable journal must be examined for validity and the relevance that it has to the topic area.

2 You may interpret the term 'critical appraisal' to mean that **you must criticize and find fault** with everything that you read. Often the term critical is interpreted to mean that unless you 'tear to pieces' what you find, then you have not done your job. Although it is always possible to find faults with every piece of research, it needs to be remembered that no research is perfect. Therefore when you look for strengths and weaknesses remember to take a balanced approach. More credible authors may identify within their own methodology what they consider to be any weaknesses with their approach.

Access some research from a professional journal and see if you can identify any critical comment on the paper.

Many journals offer a review of the paper alongside the article or in the next edition. Try and spot how a reviewer offers both positive and negative comments on the paper.

How do you identify if you have got a research paper or review of research?

It is important that you identify what type of information you have, so that you know that you have the most appropriate information for your needs. First of all, determine whether the evidence you have is a research paper or a review of research. This is not always as easy as it sounds! Research papers begin with a research question and have a methods section followed by results then a conclusion.

If you have found a research study or review of research, this should be recognizable by having a clearly described *methods* section followed by a *results* or *findings* section. There is also likely to be an abstract which contains a summary of this information.

You may be lucky and find a recent, good quality systematic review but remember you still need to appraise it. If not, then you need to appraise and synthesize all the information you have found. At this point it is normal to feel swamped by the amount of literature and perhaps the unfamiliar terms and language used in the papers you find.

Again, refer back to Chapter 4 in this book or access another research textbook or glossary to find out more about the research methods that are used in the papers you have accessed.

There are many different types of research in health and social care and the format for describing the research and results will vary widely, however the fundamental features of describing the methods used to undertake the research and the research findings should be clearly described in all research papers. They may use the word study, review, or mention specific types of research that you may need to look up if you are unfamiliar with them. The abstract should help you to identify if the evidence you have is a research paper or not.

Example *abstract* from a research paper (Gardner *et al.* 2011: 491)

Background: This prospective, randomized, controlled clinical trial compared changes in exercise performance and daily ambulatory activity in peripheral artery disease patients with intermittent claudication after a home-based exercise program, a supervised exercise program, and usual-care control.

Methods and Results: Of the 119 patients randomized, 29 completed home-based exercises, 33 completed supervised exercise, and 30 completed usual-care control. Both exercise programs consisted of intermittent walking to nearly maximal claudication pain for 12 weeks. Patients wore a step activity monitor during each exercise session. Primary outcome measures included claudication onset time and peak walking time obtained from a treadmill exercise test; secondary outcome measures included daily ambulatory cadences measured during a 7-day monitoring period. Adherence to home-based and supervised exercise was similar ($p = 0.712$) and exceeded 80%. Both exercise programs increased claudication onset time ($p < 0.001$) and peak walking time ($p < 0.01$), whereas only home-based exercise increased daily average cadence ($p < 0.01$). No changes were seen in the control group ($p > 0.05$). The changes in claudication onset time and peak walking time were similar between the 2 exercise groups ($p > 0.05$), whereas the change in daily average cadence was greater with home-based exercise ($p < 0.05$).

Conclusions: A home-based exercise program, quantified with a step activity monitor, has high adherence and is efficacious in improving claudication measures similar to a standard supervised exercise program. Furthermore, home-based exercise appears more efficacious in increasing daily ambulatory activity in the community setting than supervised exercise.

You can see from this abstract that the paper is a research paper, reporting the findings of a randomized controlled trial. However it is not always so easy to recognize a piece of research. For example, bear the following points in mind:

- Beware news reports of research published in the news section of journals (or the national television news) that just show headline 'high impact' findings but omit all other findings. This report is not a full report of the research but is reported on by a journalist, who may have cherry picked what he wanted to report on. Try to obtain the original research paper.
- Beware academic writing that refers to lots of research and resembles a review of research but does not tell you how the review was assembled. If you cannot see a methods section telling you how the review was undertaken, then you are probably not looking at a good quality literature review.

If you have identified research, Greenhalgh (2010) states that there are **three preliminary questions** to get you started in critical appraisal:

Q. 1. What was the research question – and why was the study needed?
The first sentence of a research paper should state clearly the background. For example, *'It is widely known that . . . however. . . there is a lack of clear evidence that . . .'*. There should then be a brief literature review to show awareness of what has been done on the topic.

Q. 2. What was the research design?
You should assess if the paper is reporting from primary *(they did their own research)* or secondary sources *(they are reporting or summarizing other studies)*.

Q. 3. Was the research design appropriate to the question?

We have discussed this in detail in Chapter 4 where we refer to the concept of 'hierarchies of evidence' and how certain types of research suit certain research questions. We also refer to the concept of developing 'your own hierarchy of evidence' (Aveyard 2010) for the information needs that you have. The main point to re-emphasize is that there is no one 'hierarchy of evidence' and it depends on what you need to find out.

Fineout-Overholt *et al.* (2010) in the fifth article in a series on evidence-based practice describe **rapid critical appraisal** as reviewing each study initially to determine the level of evidence, how well it was conducted and how useful it is to practice. They suggest using the relevant hierarchy of evidence to help determine the level of the evidence, a relevant critical appraisal tool to determine how well it is conducted, and they suggest an **evaluation table to summarize each paper** and help decide its usefulness. See http://download.lww.com/wolterskluwer_vitalstream_com/PermaLink/AJN/A/AJN_110_7_2010_07_27_AJN_0_SDC1.pdf. We offer an alternative table later in this chapter.

If you are wondering if the evidence is research or a review of research but you cannot see a methods and results section, then it probably isn't!

You may find it useful to use a research textbook or glossary to look up any methods or research types you are unfamiliar with – or ask someone! You could use a health or social care **dictionary** or online **glossary**, some publishers offer useful glossaries or specialist groups such as this site for social workers funded by the Social Care Institute for Excellence (SCIE) (http://www.resmind.swap.ac.uk/content/00_other/glossary.htm). Cochrane also has a glossary (http://www.cochrane.org/glossary/5).

How do you identify if you have got a discussion or opinion paper?

Discussion or opinion papers will not have the same structure as a research paper and will generally be introduced as representing the opinion of the author. Sometimes however there is no such introduction and the aim of the paper might be harder to find. You need to read the paper closely to ascertain what the aim and purpose of the paper is. Remember that however authoritative the writer sounds, if he or she is only expressing an opinion this evidence remains anecdotal.

It is quite common to find informative papers which give a general update about a topic. They are often written up in an 'essay' style. At first glance you might think that you have found a literature review, because these papers often refer to lots of research, however if you look closely, these papers will not have a methods section to say how they found their literature. It can be confusing to identify whether such updates have been compiled using a systematic and unbiased approach or not.

In principle, if the paper does not include a specific question and a method recounting how the update was put together, you should not consider this to be a comprehensive review.

This will provide less strong evidence than a review which has been compiled systematically. Remember that the quality of this type of evidence will depend on the person writing the paper. They can be very useful but do not assume that an expert is using relevant evidence-based sources upon which to base his or her argument. There may be bias in the selection of the sources used.

Example *abstract* from a paper that is not a systematic review or research paper:

'Mental health problems are common in older people admitted to general hospitals. With an increasing ageing population, admissions will rise and nurses will be expected to manage patients' co-existing mental health problems as well as physical problems. This article explores potential strategies for the management of patients with depression, delirium and dementia. The emphasis is on improving quality of care for this group of vulnerable patients' (Keenan *et al.* 2011: 46).

Getting to know your literature

The next thing to do is to **become familiar** with the literature you have got.

Read and **re-read** the material so that you become familiar with it. Check that you are confident that you know which type of evidence you have: research, discussion or other evidence. At this point, you should be able to discuss with confidence the content of your papers.

Read a study or review and see if you can discuss it in detail with someone else without referring back to the papers or at least with minimal reference!

Relevance of the research

Making sense of each individual paper you come across is therefore very important and will enable you to make important assessments as to the relevance of the paper to your topic of study in addition to identifying the strengths and limitations – and therefore the impact that the paper will have on addressing what you are trying to find out.

At first glance, a research paper might appear to address your research question directly, however on closer inspection you realize that the scope of the paper is very different from what your initial assessment had led you to believe and in fact has only indirect relevance to your research question.

You might find that although the context of the paper is relevant to your research question, the methods used in the paper have been poorly carried out and you are less confident in the results of the study as a result.

Group your literature together so that you have all the qualitative research papers in one pile, the quantitative papers in another, discussion and opinion in another and so on. Be aware that some may comprise mixed methods. When you have done this, you will be able to **select the correct appraisal tool** for the type of research you have identified.

Overall, you may find several studies of just one type of research or you might have a combination of qualitative and quantitative research, maybe some systematic reviews and other non-research information, such as discussion and opinion articles.

Activity: you may want to organize a table or index cards to help you sort out the information you have. Consider using colour highlighters or *Post-it* notes to help with this. ***Fill in what you can at first*** and then as you develop your appraisal skills you can add more.

You may find a **table format** helpful where you can **summarize** what you have found. See the example below or the online **evaluation table** by Fineout-Overholt *et al.* (2010) (http://download.lww.com/wolterskluwer_vitalstream_com/PermaLink/AJN/A/AJN_110_7_2010_07_27_AJN_0_SDC1.pdf). If you have been working through this book systematically, you should be able to fill in all the categories except the strengths and weaknesses, which we come to at the next stage of this chapter:

Authors names	Aims of review/study or research question	Journal	Type of evidence	Strengths	Limitations	Main findings
Smith and Brown (2007)	They have 3 clear objectives . . .	Journal of applied social work – peer reviewed	Systematic review	Clear methodology Good quality studies . . .	It is 6 years old and things may have changed	They found that . . .
Chin and Chan (2010)	Vague statement . . . differs from the abstract	International journal of physiotherapy	Randomized Controlled Trial	Good sample size, wide range of participants	Don't discuss ethical issues/ consent or how they carried out blinding	Clear statistical significance in main finding statement . . .

Table 6.1 Sample table for helping you summarize the papers identified by your search

In the next section we discuss the use of critical appraisal tools in more detail. It is important to note that before you use a tool, you need to be familiar with the research approach that you come across. A critical appraisal tool will not help you understand the research used in the paper – it merely prompts you to ask relevant questions of the paper. **Before** you appraise a paper, **you need to be familiar with the research methodology** used in that paper. Therefore if you are uncertain as to what constitutes good quality research for a particular research method, read more widely about that particular research approach.

General critical appraisal tools

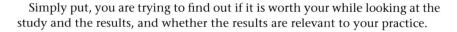

Critical appraisal tools are *checklists* to help you ask questions of the evidence you have in order to assist you in determining *how strong* and *how relevant* the evidence is.

Simply put, you are trying to find out if it is worth your while looking at the study and the results, and whether the results are relevant to your practice.

- Critical appraisal tools help you develop a **consistent** approach to the critique of research and other information.
- They **only help** with the critical appraisal – they do not do the work for you! If you do not understand the methods by which the research has been undertaken, the tool will not help you. Therefore you need to understand **what impacts on the quality and relevance** for each type of research you use so that you can appraise it. Some general reading about research methods will help with this.
- When you use a paper as evidence it is important to **judge** its quality, not just report what the paper says.

Benefits and cautions when using an appraisal tool

The review process is complex and use of an appraisal tool will assist in the development of a systematic approach to this process and ensure that all papers are reviewed with equal rigour. Critical appraisal tools will guide you through questions you need to ask of each type of paper you have. Some tools ask questions that if used simplistically, can result in the appraiser **just reporting** what the paper says rather than forming a judgement. Anyone can report the findings of a paper. It takes more skill to make a judgement as to the value of the results. This is where it is important that as an appraiser you have a good understanding of what factors influence quality in the different types of research.

However, before you reach for an appraisal tool, a note of caution has been issued by Katrak *et al.* (2004) and more recently by Crowe and Sheppard (2011) who demonstrate that whilst there are many appraisal tools that are easily available, there are few studies of the rigour and usefulness of the appraisal tools themselves. In their paper, Crowe and Sheppard (2011) conclude that users of appraisal tools should be careful about which tool they use and how they use it as there is an absence of strong evidence about the rigour of the tools themselves. In another study, Dixon-Woods *et al.* (2007) carried out a study to compare the way in which experienced researchers appraised a number of papers using three appraisal methods – unprompted judgement, or one of two appraisal tools. They concluded that the structured approach of the appraisal tools did not produce greater consistency of judgements about the quality of papers. However, the participants in this research were experienced researchers and, despite the notes of caution expressed, we would recommend the use of appraisal tools for those new to research and its evaluation.

Starting with a general appraisal tool

There are a vast number of critical appraisal tools available. A quick search engine search (such as Google) will enable you to identify a good many, others can be found in research or study skills textbooks and research or evidence-based practice journals.

For those starting out with critical appraisal, we recommend our '**six questions to trigger critical thinking**' appraisal tool (Aveyard *et al.* 2011: 15). This tool has been developed for use with any piece of evidence and prompts the user to consider aspects of EBP we consider throughout this book.

Six questions to trigger critical thinking	
Where did you find the information? Did you just 'come across' it? Or did you access it through a systematic search?	**What** is it and **what** are the key messages or results/findings? Is it a research study, professional opinion, discussion, website or other?
How has the author/speaker come to their conclusions? Is their line of reasoning logical and understandable? If it is research or a review of research, how was it carried out, was it done well, and do the conclusions reflect the findings?	**Who** has written/said this? Is the author/speaker an organization or individual? Are they an expert in the topic? Could they have any bias? How do you know?
When was this written/said? Older key information may still be valid, but you need to check if there had been more recent work.	**Why** has this been written/said? Who is the information aimed at – professionals or patient/client groups? What is the aim of the information?

Some notes about our appraisal tool:

1 **Where did you find the information?** The purpose of this question is to emphasize the importance of undertaking a comprehensive search for evidence rather than relying on 'ad hoc' methods. When a thorough search is not undertaken, you cannot be sure that you are getting a representative sample of literature on which to base your academic work or clinical or professional practice.

2 **What is it and what are the key messages/results/ findings?** The purpose of this question is to emphasize the importance of recognizing the type of evidence that you have. Research is generally stronger evidence than non-research papers and it is important to be able to recognize what you have. If it is not primary research or a review, you need to judge the quality of the arguments or evidence presented. If you hear about some evidence try and find out where the information came from. It is important to summarize the findings.

3 **How has the author/speaker come to their conclusions?** The purpose of this question is to emphasize the importance of being critical of the methods used in a paper – whether it is a research or discussion paper – so that you can form an idea about the validity of the conclusions. If someone is presenting a verbal argument, what are they basing it on?

4 **Who has written/said this/where is it published/presented?** For written sources, it is important to consider the journal of publication, and in written and spoken sources of information **consider the expertise of the authors.** In principle, a journal is considered to be of good quality if it is **peer reviewed** – that is, each paper is reviewed by at least one recognized expert in the subject area about which the paper is written prior to acceptance for publication in the journal.

Remember: peer review is not perfect!

It is not uncommon for corrections or amendments to a paper to appear in later publications of the journal. In reality, the peer review process takes place when the research paper is published! As a general rule, just as you may be more likely to take an argument more seriously if it is published in one newspaper rather than another, this is also the case with academic journals. You should consider whether or not the authors include their relevant qualifications and have the experience to write or speak authoritatively on the topic. For research it is also particularly important that they have the necessary experience to undertake the research.

Access a journal's website for an overview of its publishing process and ask educationalists/senior colleagues what are considered high quality journals in your profession.

5 **When was it written/said?** Older information may be valid but you need to check if there has been more recent work. Is there anything more recent that has disagreed with or supported what they write or say?

6 **Why has this been written/said?** Who is the information aimed at? Is it for specific practitioners or client/patient groups? If it is a research paper, the study question should be clear and should be founded on an argument and a rationale as to why the study was undertaken (background and context). If it is a discussion paper, the authors should state this early on in the paper. Might the authors or speakers have their own agenda or interests (i.e. involvement in any commercial, financial or other areas of potential bias?)

The purpose of our **Six Questions to Trigger Critical Thinking** is that it provides a generic tool that can be used on any evidence that you find and helps you to identify the type of evidence that you have.

Additional general critical appraisal tools

Other 'general' checklists are available to help you evaluate the evidence you come across and to think critically about arguments and evidence. These include Cottrell (2011). There are more sources given in Chapter 7 and in our useful websites section. A website called 'netting the evidence' has developed a search engine dedicated to the methodology of evidence-based practice (available at http://tinyurl.com/2poh3a). This makes searching for checklists etc. much more focussed.

Crowe and Sheppard (2011) have developed a critical appraisal tool that can be used with a variety of research types. It has **eight main categories:**

1 Preamble
2 Introduction
3 Design
4 Sampling
5 Data collection
6 Ethical matters
7 Results
8 Discussion.

Each category has a description and the appraiser can score between 1 and 5 in each category. There is a user guide to the scoring system available. It has been evaluated, albeit by the authors, for its validity (Crowe *et al.* 2012: 377). They reported that it should reflect a true assessment of the research.

Greenhalgh (2010) includes general checklists in the appendices of her book (in addition to the specific checklists we discuss later). She recommends that readers ask questions to determine **what the study is about, what type of study it is,** whether or not the **design is appropriate** and whether or not it meets, the **expected standards of ethics and quality.**

Various **text books** or **overview articles** on research methods and evidence-based practice will also offer appraisal tools – it is worth looking in your local library or if possible accessing e-books so you can search online for specific tools. There is an excellent series of 12 articles called 'Evidence-based practice step by step' in the *American Journal of Nursing* 2010 – all are accessible on the internet (http://journals.lww.com/ajnonline/pages/collectiondetails.aspx?TopicalCollectionId=10).

Specific critical appraisal tools

If you need to use a more detailed tool, it is probably most useful to use a *specific critical appraisal tool* (sometimes abbreviated as CATs) *that is relevant* to the type of research you are using.

If you have already had some experience of critical appraisal, you might want to start with a more specific critical appraisal tool which focusses on a specific research methodology. Appraisal tools which are specifically focussed on the type of research paper you have will contain questions which are closely related to the specific study design in question, providing an appropriate structure for the review. Many critical appraisal tools have been developed for the review of specific types of research, and as such are **design specific**, for example, for the review of randomized controlled trials only.

There are many sources of critical appraisal tools, from specific professional groups, disciplines and academic and clinical institutions. It is worth searching to see if you can find one that you like, or is relevant (check the date and authors too). Here are a few examples, there are more in Chapter 7 and in our **'useful websites'** at the end of this book:

Critical Appraisal Tools

One of the most widely used sets of appraisal tools are from the **Critical Appraisal Skills Programme** (CASP International Network 2010). They have produced critical appraisal tools for the appraisal of many different types of research including RCTs, systematic reviews, cohort and case control studies and qualitative studies. They are available at: http://www.caspinternational.org/

The Oxford based **Centre for Evidence-Based Medicine** (CEBM) has different appraisal tools for systematic reviews, RCTs, diagnostic and prognosis studies available at: http://www.cebm.net/index.aspx?o=1157

An Introduction to Evidence-Informed Public Health and A Compendium of Critical Appraisal Tools for Public Health Practice available at: http://www.empho.org.uk/Download/Public/11615/1/CA%20Tools%20for%20Public%20Health.pdf

The **Scottish Intercollegiate Guidelines Network** (SIGN) which brings together evidence-based guidelines has a range of appraisal checklists available at http://sign.ac.uk/methodology/checklists.html

This site offers a variety of checklists from **Glasgow University** http://www.gla.ac.uk/researchinstitutes/healthwellbeing/research/generalpractice/ebp/checklists/#d.en.19536

As a novice appraiser and at undergraduate level, you may initially consider the main questions only, and only when you are more experienced or more widely read consider the additional more detailed questions. Those studying at postgraduate level might want to refer to these more detailed questions. You are likely to need access to a research textbook or dictionary to look up what you don't understand. As with all appraisal tools, when considering your answers to each of the CASP questions, you will need to evaluate the study (not just describe it). Remember you are judging the quality of the study. To do this, you will need to think carefully about what the authors have not said in their article, as well as what they have written.

One of us, in another publication, (Sharp and Taylor 2012) developed some **prompt questions** to help you use two of the CASP appraisal tools; one for RCTs and one for qualitative research (adapted from CASP International 2010 and presented under each method below). We developed these as we found that when they were just using the CASP questions, our students were just describing what was in the papers they were reviewing, rather than evaluating them, or giving reasons why the issues they commented on mattered. The prompt questions might be useful to help you think critically but are not an exhaustive list of things you should consider, just some suggestions to get you started. They only apply to the **RCTs** and **Qualitative research CASP tools** and you should note that other tools may be best for the type of research you have found.

Key questions to ask when reviewing different types of evidence

We will now discuss the **key questions** you should ask of the different types of evidence you are likely to encounter and provide some examples of critical appraisal tools you might find useful. Remember you can look at the specific tools and prompt questions if relevant. The different types of evidence are:

- Review articles
- Quantitative studies
- Qualitative studies
- Professional and clinical guidelines and policy
- Non-research information, for example discussion and opinion or anecdotal evidence
- Websites.

Key questions to ask of review articles and good quality literature reviews

We have discussed the value of systematic reviews and good quality literature reviews in detail throughout this book. We suggest the following questions should be asked to determine if the review is of good quality.

Has the review been undertaken systematically?

Those evaluating review articles should be able to determine whether the review was undertaken in an explicit systematic way or whether a more haphazard and random approach has been used. A review incorporating a systematic approach will present stronger evidence than a review that does not.

Are the researchers explicit about the methods used to achieve this review?

You should check if the authors have said clearly how they undertook the review, what terms they used, over what period, how they decided what to include etc.? The amount of detail given to the search, critiquing and bringing together of the evidence will differ with each literature review. You should scrutinize the methods used to conduct the review.

Do the researchers demonstrate that they did everything in their power to ensure their approach was as systematic as possible? If the review is described as a **Cochrane or Campbell Collaboration review** you can be fairly confident that it is a review that has been undertaken systematically. There is a handbook that guides such reviews to ensure consistency (http://www.cochrane.org/training/cochrane-handbook or http://www.campbellcollaboration.org/resources/research/the_production.php).

> **Example:** a Cochrane-style systematic review aims to uncover **all literature** on the topic in question. It will have a team of researchers, who work together with explicit criteria in the selection and critical analysis of the literature.

A less detailed review is likely to be carried out by a single researcher with fewer resources for collaboration in these aspects. A less detailed review will acknowledge that the search is unlikely to be exhaustive but is likely to **identify the databases used.**

See if you can find a systematic review relating to your profession using a database or from the Cochrane website (www.cochrane.org), or Campbell collaboration (http://www.campbellcollaboration.org/).

Examples of critical appraisal tools of review articles

One of the critical appraisal tools for the appraisal of a systematic review is the CASP tool for systematic reviews http://www.caspinternational.org/?o=1012 and you can find one at the Centre for Evidence Based Medicine (CEBM) http://www.cebm.net/index.aspx?o=1157

Key questions to ask of quantitative studies

In Chapter 4, we have described two main approaches to quantitative studies – experimental and non-experimental.

Using a database, see if you can find a quantitative study relating to your profession.

The key questions of quantitative research you need to ask are outlined next.

What method was selected to undertake the research?

In most papers there will be a short summary of the research process undertaken and from this you will be able to identify how the study was conducted. Make sure you understand the method.

How big was the sample size?

The sample refers to the number who took part in the study. The authors of quantitative research papers should demonstrate how they determined the sample size for the research in question. This should be clearly documented in the paper and is often referred to as a **power calculation.**

The power calculation is a statistical test undertaken by those designing the research study in order to ensure that the sample used in the research is big enough for the findings to be considered reliable.

> **For example:** the findings of a small study are likely to be less reliable than those of a larger study as they may be due to chance variations. With a larger sample, the findings are less likely to be due to chance.

Has the appropriate sample been obtained?

You need to ask yourself, **who was selected to participate** in the study? Quantitative research sometimes uses **random sampling.** This means that the sample is picked at random from the overall population. When you are reviewing a quantitative study, be aware of the sampling strategy and be able to comment on the reasons as to why this approach has been adopted. Consider whether a random or non-random sample was used and whether this was appropriate.

How were the data collected?

The data collection method should be **appropriate** for the study design. Quantitative research often uses a wide range of data collection methods that are appropriate for objective measurement such as survey/ questionnaires, objective physiological tests, observation, and rates of occurrence (incidence). *Notice how researchers say the data were collected (not was collected).*

How were the data analysed?

Quantitative data are usually analysed statistically and you should expect to find reference to the statistical tests used in the paper in order to make sense of the data. There should be numerical presentation of the data and discussion of these findings. You might expect to see such terms as **confidence intervals** and **statistical significance** including **p value** discussed. There will probably be a section entitled **main findings/results.** You should consider if the data analysis is **objective.**

Resources for those reviewing RCTs

Sharp and Taylor adapted the CASP International Network (2010) tool to come up with this list of prompt tools for evaluating RCTs:

Prompt questions to help you evaluate rather than just report (Sharp and Taylor (2012) adapted from CASP International Network (2010) tool for RCTs)

1. Did the trial address a clearly focussed issue?
☐ Did they ask a question, or state an aim?
   Tip: a question should have a question mark (?) at the end of it.
☐ Why is it important to have a clearly focussed question or stated aim?

2. Was the assignment of patients to treatments randomized?
☐ How were participants allocated? Was it truly random?
☐ Was there any bias?
☐ Were the two groups equal in all respects? Did the researchers consider the essential characteristics (variables) of their sample and control for them?
☐ What are the implications of the randomization process they used for the results of *this* study?

3. Were all of the participants who entered the trial properly accounted for at its conclusion?
☐ Was intention-to-treat analysis undertaken?
☐ Why is it important for *this* study's findings?
☐ Why is 'loss to follow up' important for this study's findings?

4. Were participants, health workers and study personnel 'blind' to treatments?
☐ Was double or single blinding achieved? Why? Was this an appropriate choice?
☐ What are the implications of their approach to blinding for the results of *this* study?

5. Were the groups similar at the start of the trial?
☐ Were the groups matched in terms of age, sex, location etc., or was stratified randomization used?
☐ Is this important for this study and why?

6. Aside from the experimental intervention, were the groups treated equally?
☐ How were the groups followed up?
☐ Were there any differences in how the groups were followed up and would it make any difference to the results of this study?

7. How large was the treatment effect?
☐ What was the difference in outcomes between the control and experimental group?
☐ Was a power calculation conducted?
☐ What are the implications of their sample size for the results of *this* study?

8. How precise was the estimate of the treatment effect?
☐ Are there any inconsistencies (or errors) between the statistics presented and the discussion or conclusions drawn?

☐ Are the results statistically significant? What does this mean?
☐ Did they use p values and confidence intervals/limits, why is this useful?

9. Can the results be applied to the local population?
☐ *Are the participants similar to your own?*
☐ *Do any differences matter? If so why?*

10. Were all clinically important outcomes considered?
☐ What did they not consider that might have influenced the results?
☐ Overall is this study of good enough quality to be useful?
☐ Given all the points you have made above, how generalizable are the results?
☐ Is further research needed?

11. Are the benefits worth the harms and costs?
☐ Is the intervention worth adopting in practice and policy? What do you think based on your appraisal?
☐ Is it too expensive to adopt?
☐ Are the side effects/or any harms worth it?

In addition to the specific CASP appraisal tools for Randomized Controlled Trials available at http://www.caspinternational.org/?o=1012, there are further resources for those reviewing quantitative studies.

The CONSORT (Consolidated Standards of Reporting Trials) (CONSORT 2010) have produced the **CONSORT Statement** available at http://www.consort-statement.org/ which is an evidence-based, minimum set of recommendations for reporting RCTs. It offers a standard way for authors to prepare reports of trial findings, facilitating their complete and transparent reporting, and aiding their critical appraisal and interpretation. Full details of the CONSORT statement are given by Schulz *et al.* (2011).

Resources for those reviewing cohort studies and case controlled studies

There is the **Newcastle-Ottawa Scale for assessing the quality of non-randomized studies in meta-analyses** (no date) including cohort studies and case control studies (available at http://www.ohri.ca/programs/clinical_epidemiology/oxford.asp). There is also the CASP critical appraisal tool for cohort studies and case controlled studies (http://www.caspinternational.org/?o=1012) and SIGN (http://www.sign.ac.uk/methodology/checklists.html).

Resources for those reviewing survey/questionnaires

On one level, surveys and questionnaires are easy to critique as we are all so familiar with the method of research. It is unlikely that anyone reading this book has not completed a questionnaire or survey at some point and also formed an opinion as to the relevance of the questionnaire which may have ended up in the bin rather than back in the researcher's office! There have been few appraisal tools for questionnaires/surveys and they are often poorly devised. CASP and CEBM do not offer appraisal tools for questionnaires.

Can you think of a time when you have found a questionnaire hard to answer or when the meaning of the questions has been unclear?

We have simplified Greenhalgh's (2010) detailed checklist below to provide you with some good questions to ask when reviewing questionnaires and surveys:

1 Is a questionnaire the best way to find out the information?
2 Is there already a validated questionnaire available and did they use it, if not why?
3 Have the authors discussed the reliability and validity of the questionnaire?
4 Was a pilot study of the questionnaire carried out and amended if need be?
5 Was the sample size big enough and did it represent the population group adequately?
6 Was the questionnaire distributed and administered in an appropriate way?
7 Were issues such as literacy levels, language etc. considered?
8 Was the response rate high? If not, have the researchers discussed any potential differences between those who responded and those who didn't and the impact on the results?
9 Was the data analysis appropriate?
10 What were the results? Were they statistically significant and all results including negative ones reported?
11 If there were qualitative responses have they been reported and interpreted adequately and have qualitative data (e.g. free text responses) been adequately and reasonably presented?
12 Have the researchers realistically presented a link between the data presented and their conclusions?

The next time you find a questionnaire, or are asked to complete one, try and critically appraise it using some of the principles outlined above.

Key questions to ask of qualitative studies

There has been much discussion in recent years concerning the ways in which qualitative research is evaluated and this debate is on-going.

This is because there is often no set approach or standard for carrying out qualitative research and methods are being developed all the time – therefore it is difficult to evaluate it.

Most qualitative researchers argue that it is not possible to assess qualitative research in the same way as quantitative research. For this reason, researchers such as Lincoln and Guba (1985) have long since argued that the **following terms are more appropriate** for to assessing the quality of a qualitative study than terms such as validity and reliability:

- **Credibility** – do the findings ring true from the approach taken? Are they well presented and meaningful?
- **Transferability** – can the results be transferred into a different setting?
- **Dependability** – can you rely on the results as they are presented?
- **Confirmability** – could the study be repeated?

See if you can identify a qualitative research study by accessing a database and looking at the titles and abstracts.

Overall, when critiquing qualitative literature, remember that critical appraisal of qualitative research is complex. Those reviewing qualitative research should become familiar with the particular approaches to qualitative study that have been used in the papers they have identified.

The key questions of qualitative research you need to ask are:

Was a qualitative method appropriate?

Consider whether a qualitative method was appropriate for the study and specifically whether in-depth exploration was the best way to collect data for this study.

Who was the sample?

You would expect to see purposive, theoretical, convenience or snowball sampling. Do the researchers give a clear rationale for their sampling approach? What type of participant makes up the purposive sample and are they the most relevant?

How big was the sample?

You would expect the sample size to be large enough to achieve sufficient information-rich cases for in-depth data analysis, but not so large that the amount of data obtained becomes unmanageable. Has the way in which the sample size was arrived at been clearly explained?

How were the data collected?

It is important that the researchers justify the approach they have taken to the data collection process and can demonstrate that the process was undertaken systematically and rigorously. The way of collecting the actual data should also be appropriate to the method and research question. Most researchers agree that in-depth **interviews and focus groups** should be tape recorded so that the interviews can be **transcribed** (an exact word-for-word account of what was said). However, some researchers argue that this is time consuming and that the time could be better used by undertaking additional interviews and hence collecting considerably more data.

Is a rationale given for data collection?

Is the reason for **interviews or focus groups** clearly stated? Focus groups are a form of group interview and may be selected over in-depth interviews when dialogue **between research participants** is considered beneficial. If the research topic is unfamiliar to those involved and participants may not have developed their thoughts in relation to this topic, focus groups can be useful as a data collection method as the ideas expressed by one participant may trigger a response in another participant. Ask yourself whether the researchers have considered the disadvantages (limitations) of the approaches used?

> **Example:** if a topic is particularly sensitive, participants may be reluctant to express their thoughts in a focus group and in-depth interviews may be more appropriate.

Questionnaires might be used in the collection of **qualitative data**. Whilst it is possible to collect qualitative data through open ended questions on a questionnaire schedule, such data is not likely to be as in depth as that collected through one to one interaction.

Observational data may be used in both quantitative and qualitative studies if researchers want to see what people actually do rather than what they say they do. Data collected through **observation** is especially useful for this. If the observed activity is counted then this would be quantitative, and if described and interpreted, then this would be a qualitative approach. For example the number of infection control practices undertaken by each practitioner could be counted numerically, or the nature of the interaction between practitioner and patient could be observed using qualitative approaches. Researchers need to consider the **Hawthorne effect** which refers to the tendency of people who are observed to behave differently (usually better) than they would usually (Eckmanns *et al.* 2006).

Who collected the data?

Is the interviewer **trained and skilled** in asking questions that probe into the experience of the participant and is the aim clearly stated in order to generate rich data through one to one dialogue?

How was the data analysed?

Word restrictions impose limitations on the detail that can be given in any journal paper, but there should be evidence of a considered approach to data analysis. Did more than one person try and independently code the data or identify the themes?

Has a computer package been used to analyse the data?

This in itself does not ensure rigour in the analysis process, but you might expect to see some acknowledgement of the possibilities for data analysis using different methods. It is possible to demonstrate rigour in data analysis without the use of computer packages.

Is there justification as to how much data had been collected?

The researchers should seek to justify how many interviews or focus groups or other forms of qualitative data they collected.

Was data saturation achieved?

Data saturation means that at the end of the analysis period, the continuing data analysis does not identify additional new themes from the data, but instead the data that is analysed merely adds to the existing themes that have emerged from previous data analysis.

Resources for those reviewing qualitative studies

You should then assess the rigour of the papers with the aid of a critical appraisal tool. There is a CASP tool for qualitative research: http://www.caspinternational.org/?o=1012. See also the **prompt questions offered here:**

Prompt questions to help you evaluate rather than just report
(Sharp and Taylor (2012) adapted from CASP International Network (2010) tool for qualitative studies).

Look at the front page of CASP tool and the sub-questions too!

1. Was there a clear statement of the aims of the research?
☐ Did they ask a question, or state an aim?
Tip: a question should have a question mark (?) at the end of it.

2. Is a qualitative methodology appropriate?
☐ How does this study reflect the key characteristics of qualitative research?
☐ Given the aim of *this* study, why is qualitative research more appropriate than quantitative research?

3. Was the research design appropriate to address the aims of the research?
☐ What are the advantages/limitations of this study's design compared to another design they might have considered?
☐ Do the advantages of their chosen design outweigh the limitations in order to achieve their research aims? Why?
☐ How does the design they chose impact on their research findings?

4. Was the recruitment strategy appropriate to the aims of the research?
☐ How were people recruited?
☐ What sampling strategy was used? How did the researchers define and justify the strategy that they used?
☐ What are the advantages/disadvantages of this strategy for *this* study's aims?
☐ Is there anything that the researchers overlooked?
☐ Was the sampling strategy biased? If so, what sort of bias?
☐ What are the implications of this for the findings of *this* study?

5. Were the data collected in a way that addressed the research issues?
☐ How was the data collected?
☐ Why was this method of data collection *particularly* useful for this study's aims?
☐ Were alternatives considered?
☐ Is there anything that the researchers overlooked?
☐ What are the implications of this for *this* study's findings?

6. Has the relationship between researcher and participants been adequately considered?
☐ What was the relationship?
☐ Was reflexivity discussed? What is this? What purpose does it serve?
☐ Did this study demonstrate reflexivity?

☐ How did the researchers enable/restrict the participants' ability to talk about their experiences on this topic?

☐ What might they have overlooked?

☐ What are the implications for *this* study's findings?

7. Have ethical issues been taken into account?

☐ What ethical issues did they consider?

☐ Which ethical principles did they recognize? What are these principles and how are they defined?

☐ Is there anything that the researchers overlooked?

☐ Might there have been any coercion? Or bias?

☐ What are the implications for the findings of *this* study?

8. Was the data analysis sufficiently rigorous?

☐ How did they analyse the data?

☐ Given their chosen design, was this appropriate?

☐ Did they do all they could to ensure that data analysis was rigorous?

☐ Did they use respondent validation (member checking)? What is this? How necessary is it for their research design?

☐ Is there anything that the researchers overlooked?

☐ How do they demonstrate trustworthiness?

☐ What are the implications for the findings of *this* study?

9. Is there a clear statement of findings?

☐ What are the findings?

☐ Do the findings clearly and accurately emerge from the data?

10. How valuable is the research?

☐ Think about the purpose of qualitative research findings. Now consider all the points you have made above regarding the rigour and validity of this study, and evaluate how useful the study's findings are for practice.

We have also simplified Greenhalgh's (2010) **checklist for qualitative research below:**

1 Is the context and importance of the problem clearly stated in the form of a question? *(See information on PICOT questions in Chapter 5.)*

2 Was the specific qualitative approach appropriate?

3 How were the place for the research and the participants *chosen? (See discussion on sample selection and size in qualitative research below.)*

4 What was the researcher's perspective/involvement, and has this been taken into account and described? *(Look up reflexive/reflexivity.)*

5 Has the researcher described their data collection methods in detail? *(See data collection discussed below.)*

6 How did they analyse the data to ensure that it was rigorous and at a high standard?
7 Are the results credible, and if so, are they relevant and significant to practice?
8 Are the conclusions drawn clearly from the results?
9 Are the findings of the study transferable to other settings? *(See definition above.)*

Key questions to ask of professional and clinical guidance and policy

As with any publication, professional and clinical guidance and policy vary in quality and should be appraised. As we have already stated, ideally, these guidelines and policy documents should be **based on the best available evidence.** However, it is still up to you to ensure that the advice given in the protocol is up to date and useful. In fact this should be the first question you ask of the guidelines or policy. Make a decision that from now on, you will ask yourself questions about the validity of the guidelines or policies you have to work with, rather than just accepting this at face value.

The Agree Collaboration offers guidance for the development of guidelines and also a **critical appraisal tool for assessing the quality of guidelines and policy.** This AGREE 11 tool (Agree Collaboration 2009) is available at http://www.agreecollaboration.org/

The National Institute of Health and Clinical Excellence (NICE) has a clinical practice guidelines manual (2009) available and they are currently consulting on a 2012 version (http://www.nice.org.uk/aboutnice/howwework/developingniceclinicalguidelines/clinicalguidelinedevelopmentmethods/GuidelinesManual2009.jsp).

We have simplified Greenhalgh's (2010) checklist for guidelines below:

1 Was there any conflict of interest in the preparation and publication?
2 Are the guidelines appropriate to your topic, and do they identify the expected outcomes in terms of health and/or cost?
3 Was someone who has expertise in bringing together evidence (meta-analysis) involved?
4 Are the conclusions based on scrutiny of all the available and relevant data?
5 Do they address controversial areas such as funding and inequalities?

6   Are they valid and reliable?
7   Are they detailed, flexible and relevant to practice?
8   Are they acceptable to, affordable by and realistic for patients to adopt?
9   Do they state how they can be shared, implemented and evaluated?

Find out where professional and clinical guidelines specifically relevant to your practice might be published.

Key questions to ask of discussion or opinion articles (anecdotal evidence)

When you come across non-research based evidence it is important that you can recognize this and be equipped to assess its usefulness. Try using our **'Six questions to trigger critical thinking'** (Aveyard *et al.* 2011) to get you started on considering the quality and purpose of what you are reading.

One approach to reviewing a paper in which arguments are presented is to assess the quality of the arguments presented. This approach was originally advocated by Thouless and Thouless (1953) who discuss the use of logic in the constructed argument presented in a discussion paper. They articulate 38 **'dishonest tricks'** commonly used in an argument or written discussion, for example:

- Using emotionally charged words
- Making conclusive statements using words such as 'all' when 'some' would be more appropriate or 'never' when 'rarely' would be more appropriate
- Using selected instances or examples
- Misrepresentation of opposing arguments
- Not mentioning counter-arguments.

Does the evidence on which the arguments are founded bear scrutiny?

If the arguments are well constructed and defensible then greater weight can be given to these arguments over those that are less well prepared and constructed. You should question the use of language, the acknowledgement of alternative approaches or lines of argument, forced analogy and false credentials. Cottrell (2011) offers useful ideas on reviewing arguments in written work. It is important to remember that the expert opinion of a well-known figure in the area might be found to contradict established findings from empirical research.

Try to think about three things you will now do differently when reading professional literature.

Key questions to ask of websites

Should I believe all information contained on websites?

The answer is of course NO! There can be no doubt that the internet contains a wealth of information that may be useful for health and social care practitioners. However, as we have seen, there is also a wealth or poor quality and misleading information. It has to be acknowledged that websites are unregulated and it is possible for anybody to publish anything on an internet site. You are therefore recommended to be critical of any websites you encounter. We recommend using our **'Six questions to trigger critical thinking'** (Aveyard *et al*. 2011) to get you started.

- The web contains many hundreds of millions of pages, including everything from rigorous research to trivia and misinformation.
- Before making use of information found on the web in your academic work, you need to make sure it is of high quality.
- You should also remember that if you use information from the web in your academic work, just like printed sources those web pages must be cited in your references of any academic work or publications (see if your organization or university has a guide to referencing).

Evaluating websites

> When evaluating the quality of web resources, you could consider the following **ABC** – adapted from Howe (2001, revised 2010) – **A**ccuracy, **A**uthority, **B**ias, **B**readth and depth, **C**omparison, **C**urrency (http://www.walthowe.com/navnet/quality.html).
>
> **Accuracy** – finding 'facts' or figures quoted on the web is not automatically a guarantee that the information is accurate. Can you check the information against other sources? Does it fit with what you already know? Do the authors of the page tell you where they got the information from?
>
> **Authority** – who is providing the information, and what evidence do you have that they know what they are talking about?
>   It is not always easy to see immediately where a particular web page comes from, and an impressive-looking, whizzy web page is not necessarily a guarantee of good quality information! If you have found the page via a link or a search engine, look for a 'Home', 'Front Page', or similar icon, and follow it to try to see whether the page authors are well-known experts, and whether they provide a mission statement, 'real-world' postal address and phone number, or a bibliography of their other articles, reports or books.

Bias – as with any source of information, it is possible for a web page to appear objective, but in fact be promoting a particular standpoint. Be critical; for example, if you have found information on a particular drug, are the writers of this web page from the company that makes the drug? From a campaign group trying to get the drug banned? Or from an independent research institute?

Breadth and depth of information – how detailed is the information? What evidence is given to support it? Does it cover all relevant areas of the subject? Does the web page link to further relevant sources of information?

Currency – it is easy to assume that information on the web must be very current (up to date), but in fact there are now many pages on the web which have not been updated for years. How current does your information need to be? Does the page say when it was last updated? (If not, try checking the Properties or Page Info option in your web browser and see if a date is given.) Do all the links to other sites still work? Remember, even if the page has been updated recently, all the information may not have been checked.

Comparison with other sources – to help you have confidence in the information you find, compare it with other sources of information on the subject: published statistics, journal articles, textbooks or other websites.

There is a useful guide to **evaluating web sources** available from Oxford Brookes Library at http://www.brookes.ac.uk/library/webeval.html.

Also, remember that there are a range of pre-evaluated 'subject gateways' available on the web, where experts have searched the web for high-quality, reliable information. These will be explored more in the next chapter and are in our **'useful websites'**.

Incorporating critical appraisal into your academic writing or when debating use of evidence in practice

In this chapter so far, we have considered ways of making sense of research and non-research evidence you may encounter. Overall, the purpose of critical appraisal is to enable you to make sense of the evidence you come across. It takes you from a position of '*do not believe everything you read*' to the position in which you have the skills to assess and evaluate what you read so that you can determine the strengths and weaknesses of the evidence you encounter. It is important to remember that you need to critically appraise – make sense of – all the evidence you read, whether you are using that evidence in your practice or in your academic writing. However, when you are using evidence in your academic work, it is useful to be mindful of the following points.

- Make sure that it is clear that you have read and understood the relevance and the quality of evidence you are using.
- Remember to give information about the **type of evidence** you are using. If it is a research study, say so; if it is a discussion article, state this.
- Resist the temptation to paraphrase or quote without evaluative comment. Make sure you give the context of the evidence you use.

Example: To show the context and value of the information source

We suggest that you avoid writing: *'Jones (2009) argues that university students prefer lectures to tutorials'* (we do not know who Jones is or how Jones has reached this conclusion).

We suggest that you write instead: *'in a questionnaire study, Jones (2009) found that 70% of students preferred lectures to tutorials'.*

Or instead write: *'Jones (2009) argues that from his own experience as a student in London, there was strong feeling among his peer group that lectures were preferable to tutorials'.*

As can be seen in the example above, it is important to distinguish between a research study based on evidence, and if so what type of evidence, or merely an opinion. This is relevant whether you are debating the use of evidence in practice or in academic writing.

As a general rule, avoid writing a statement and only giving the author's name (such as 'Jones (2006) says') as the reader is completely unaware of the context of Jones work.

In summary

Once you have found your evidence, it is vital that you are able to look at it objectively and work out firstly what it is, and secondly, whether it helps you to address what you need to find out. The purpose of critical appraisal is to determine the relevance, strengths and limitations of the information collected so that you can determine how helpful the evidence is in answering your question. A study might be well carried out but not very relevant to your research question. Alternatively, a study might be very relevant to your research question but not well designed or implemented. Furthermore, discussion and expert opinion might add interesting insight to your argument, but the quality of this information also needs to be assessed.

Key points

1 The first thing to do is identify whether you have a research paper or another type of evidence.
2 You need to read and re-read your papers before you can begin to critically appraise.
3 Critical appraisal is a necessary process in determining the relevance and quality of the published information related to your research question.
4 You need to distinguish between papers that report empirical findings and those that present discussion or expert opinion only.
5 You are advised to use one of the many critical appraisal tools that are available to structure your critical appraisal.

7

How to implement evidence-based practice

Background and overview of getting more evidence into practice • The motivation, knowledge and skills needed by the individual • Organizational motivation, learning and infrastructure • Finding solutions to the problems of implementing EBP • Challenging the practice of ourselves and others • The future of evidence-based practice • In summary • Key points

In this chapter we will:

- Give an overview of the context and reality of EBP including the barriers to evidence implementation
- Explore motivational factors both organizationally and individually and some of the roles that may contribute to the implementation of evidence
- Identify the skills needed by the evidence-based practitioner and how they can develop them further
- Offer a wider range of general and specific strategies and resources to help with accessing and using evidence in the reality of practice environments
- Consider ways that we can be constructively critical of our own and others' practice
- Recognize where further research is needed in evaluating the impact of EBP approaches.

Background and overview of 'getting more evidence into practice'

In the previous chapters of this book, we have emphasized why EBP has become so important and how the influence of EBP has grown. In a society with well-informed or 'expert patients' and free and easy access to information we are more likely to be challenged and called to account for our practice decisions. Throughout this book, we have outlined the steps you need to take when you define an area for exploration, and start to search for and evaluate the evidence you find.

In a way, that was the easy bit. It was certainly the logical part. It is easy to see the relevance of EBP, and we would probably all prefer to be cared for by a practitioner who is up to date and accountable rather than a practitioner who is reliant on unreliable sources. Even searching for and evaluating the evidence is fairly straightforward once you have worked out how to do it.

Putting the evidence into practice is what really matters. Yet in a rather alarming statement, Greenhalgh (2010) claims that *a lot* of unavoidable suffering is caused by failing to implement EBP. Kitson *et al.* (2008) argue that the spread of best practice and the use of best evidence remain sporadic. It seems that EBP is not as commonplace as we would like to see. We should perhaps be more aware of this and address the implementation and uptake of evidence.

The harder part of EBP seems to be overcoming *barriers, motivating individuals* and *organizations* to adopt an *evidence practice culture*, putting this *evidence into practice* and *evaluating its effectiveness*.

The Centre for reviews and dissemination (CRD) (http://www.york.ac.uk/inst/crd/index_guidance.htm) have a handbook for those undertaking reviews and emphasize that dissemination is a planned and active process and it should not be left to chance. They emphasize:

> Simply making research available does not ensure that those who need to know about it get to know about it, or can make sense of the findings. Dissemination is vital.
>
> (p. 20)

As discussed earlier, there are several models of EBP. Most of these emphasize getting evidence into practice as a key element. Thompson *et al.* (2005) describe the final two stages of their model as:

- *Incorporating the good quality evidence into a strategy for action, using professional judgement and patient or client preference,*
- *Evaluating the effects of any decisions and action taken.*

Once we know about the evidence, we need to use it and evaluate its use in practice. Melnyk *et al.* (2010), **in their seven step model of evidence-based practice** argue that the role of motivation evaluation and dissemination of evidence are the key components of the steps needed to get evidence into practice.

1 **Cultivate a spirit of inquiry.**
2 Ask questions in PICOT format.
3 Search for the best evidence.
4 Critically appraise the evidence.
5 Integrate the evidence with your expertise and patient preferences and values.
6 **Evaluate the outcomes of the practice decisions or changes based on evidence.**
7 **Disseminate evidence-based practice results.**

Why is it difficult to put EBP into practice?

Over recent years there has been a large body of literature that has explored the problems of implementing an evidence-based approach. For example, the BARRIERS scale is a nonspecific tool for identifying general barriers to research utilization and has been the subject of a systematic literature review by Kajermo *et al.* (2010). They concluded that the scale was reliable – that people filled it in in a similar way – but they questioned its validity – that is whether it was an accurate measure of the barriers to implementing EBP. This conclusion illustrates that the implementation of EBP is a complex area to address. Kajermo *et al.* (2010) recommended that future research should look at specific barriers in the particular context of implementation rather than generally.

 Think about what might stop you personally from adopting an EBP approach.

The top 10 barriers identified by Kajermo *et al.*:

1 Lack of awareness of the research
2 Not feeling capable of evaluating the quality of the research
3 Insufficient time on the job to implement new ideas
4 Lack of time to read research

   5 Feeling a lack of authority to change things
   6 Inadequate facilities for implementation
   7 Lack of support from other staff
   8 Lack of cooperation from physicians
   9 Not being able to understand statistical information
  10 The relevant literature is not together in one place.

Identify how this relates to the issues you have identified, read the rest of this chapter and then set a goal to adopt some of the ideas that may help you to overcome some of these barriers.

Looked at broadly, these barriers relate to both individual and organizational factors. In the next section, we will consider what we can do at an individual and an organizational level to reduce these barriers to the implementation of an evidence-based approach in professional practice.

The motivation, knowledge and skills needed by the individual

One factor that has an obvious impact on the development of an evidence-based approach is the role of the individual practitioner. The individual practitioner needs to have certain motivations, knowledge and skills in order to adopt evidence-based practices. This, together with resources, infrastructures and leadership is what is most likely to result in the best outcomes for our patients/clients.

   This first step on the road to getting evidence into practice is described as **'igniting a spirit of enquiry'** (Melnyk *et al.* 2009). This is a term that implies that there may be a spark or trigger that then starts us thinking and questioning what we do!

   Melnyk *et al.* state (2009: 51) that for EBP to accelerate and thrive, practitioners must have a 'never ending spirit of enquiry' and a strong belief in EBP. Both Melnyk and Price and Harrington (2010) emphasize the importance of knowledge and skills. Price and Harrington (2010: 8) say that a knowledgeable doer is:

   someone who selects, combines, judges and uses information in order to proceed in a professional manner.

So we can conclude that practitioners need knowledge and skills in addition to curiosity and critical thinking about best practice.

What can you do to develop knowledge and skills?

To help you improve your knowledge and skills, Greenhalgh (2010) has developed a **self-assessment** to see where you have knowledge gaps. As an individual interested in EBP you could start by assessing **'where you are up to'** by using a checklist for thinking about practice situations. We have simplified this from Greenhalgh's (2010: Appendix 1) work entitled: **Is my practice evidence based? – A context-sensitive checklist for individual clinical encounters.** This really outlines the importance of thinking broadly and critically about our patient/client encounters.

Consider the following. Do you:

1 Identify and prioritize all the patient/client problem(s), including their own perspective?
2 Fully consider alternative diagnosis (not just medical ones)?
3 Deal with any additional problems and risk factors?
4 Seek best available evidence relating to the problems?
5 Fully appraise the evidence?
6 Apply valid and relevant evidence to the problems logically and intuitively?
7 Present the options to the patient in a balanced, understandable way incorporating their preferences?
8 Arrange on-going referral, evaluation, re-assessment or future care as need be?

There are tests available to measure knowledge and skills in EBP, for instance McCluskey and Bishop (2009) adapted and evaluated the Adapted Fresno Test (AFT) for occupational therapists. They found that it was useful in measuring changes in knowledge and skills of rehabilitation professionals following training and it was most useful for novice learners. The tool was used by Crabtree *et al.* (2012) to explore whether following an EBP course, skills and knowledge were improved. They found that the students did not retain the skills in practice. This illustrates that whilst we are making progress in developing knowledge and skills in EBP, there is still some way to go.

Websites that may help you learn more about EBP

Cochrane also has a site that offers many links to tutorials and tools to support EBP: http://www.cochrane.org/About%20us/Evidence-based%20health%20care/Webliography/Tutorials-tools

You may want to access specific EBP journals; there may be one specifically for your profession, or see http://www.cochrane.org/about-us/evidence-based-health-care/webliography/journals

If you use social media then there are blogs, podcasts, Wikis etc. on http://www.cochrane.org/about-us/evidence-based-health-care/webliography/social-media

---

In order to improve your skills you can also do the following:

- Discuss with your peers how confident they are in their knowledge of practice (it is likely that most will feel the same as you).
- Discuss at your performance management meeting any professional development needs you have in relation to searching for or appraising information and ensure your manager knows where you lack knowledge for your practice.
- Find out if your organization offers any training on EBP.
- Don't wait until you need the skills of EBP (for a course or a project) before you learn them. There will be greater pressure on you then.
- Ask your manager if you can go on library training sessions or have study time to do online tutorials where available. If you are a student, access the library tutorials when they are offered to develop searching skills.
- Practise searching for evidence when you write an academic assignment rather than relying on the reference list.
- Read research and/or research books or do online tutorials (above) so that you become more familiar with the language and terminology used. Use a **glossary** or thesaurus where available (e.g. http://www.medicine.ox.ac.uk/bandolier/glossary.html).
- See if there is a team member or student on placement who has more skill in searching and appraising than you and see if they can help you develop these skills.
- Have a go! Use widely available sites such as www.cochrane.org, http://www.campbellcollaboration.org/ or http://www.evidence.nhs.uk/ and just play around to see what is available.

If you are a trainer, teacher or in a professional development role you can help develop the skills, knowledge and attitude of EBP in the following ways:

- Ensure that the skills for EBP are clear in the learning outcomes of the courses.
- Introduce EBP early on in the curriculum.
- Offer regular, timetabled library skills sessions.
- Ensure that clinical/professional skills sessions have a clear rationale and relevant research is available for students.
- Invite practitioners to contribute (as facilitators or patients) in the simulated learning environment.
- Ensure that EBP is related explicitly to decision making to ensure that students are more likely to engage with it.
- Make the use of evidence and critical appraisal evident in the grading criteria and in both academic and practice-based assignments (competencies).
- Encourage students to use subject librarians and study skills support available at the university.

- Ensure that role modelling and EBP are discussed as part of practice educator update days.
- Encourage lecturers to make explicit how the research that underpins teaching is appraised (so they role model critical appraisal in their teaching).

Dawes *et al.* (2005) provide a table describing evidence for aspects of **evidence-based practice teaching and assessments** (http://www.ncbi.nlm.nih.gov/pmc/articles/PMC544887/table/T1/). In addition, they give helpful examples of ways in which these skills can be taught and assessed. Many of these have been addressed throughout this book. However, there still remains an absence of evidence that this knowing about EBP actually impacts on outcomes for our patients/clients. This evaluation of EBP is discussed later.

The important point is that promoting an evidence-based approach requires commitment and implementation at an individual level. However as Crabtree *et al.* (2012) found, individuals also need the support of the organization.

Organizational motivation, learning and infrastructure

Moving onwards from an individual perspective, we need to look at the influence of the wider organization because as individuals although we can make a difference, together with colleagues we can have a greater impact. In order for an EBP culture to exist there needs to be a desire for its success from within the whole organization – this involves motivation, organizational culture and infrastructure, leadership and the willingness to provide resources and structures that support the uptake of EBP.

Organizational culture and initiatives

Organizations need a ***culture that embraces evidence-based practices;*** including providing the support and tools that the professionals need to engage in evidence-based care (Melnyk *et al.* 2010).

Parmelli *et al.* (2011) define **organizational culture** as:

> the shared characteristics among people within the same organization. These characteristics may include: beliefs, values, norms of behaviour, routines, traditions, and sense-making.

It is widely recognized that organizational culture will influence the way in which EBP develops. In view of this, a lot of work has been done to explore what organizations can do to promote a culture of EBP. Tabak *et al.* (2012) reviewed some of the models that try to help **disseminate and implement** evidence. One of these models is the **PARiHS** (Promoting Action on Research Implementation in Health Services) model (Kitson *et al.* 2008). The main features and assumptions of the **PARiHS** framework are that:

- Evidence is varied and comes from a range of places.
- Communication, teamwork and shared values, culture and leadership are important in successful implementation.
- The skill, style and understanding of those in roles that facilitate implementation is important.

The aim of the model is that recognition of all these points might help increase the success of the implementation and evaluation of EBP within an organization.

What motivates those in the wider organization to implement an EBP approach?

Relating to motivation, it is interesting to consider how different cultures seek to influence this. In the USA, which has, of course, a different health-care system to the UK, Melnyk *et al.* (2009) describe how **financial benefits** are being offered to increase the update of EBP and guidelines, and financial penalties are introduced where preventable injuries or infections occur. They note however that such factors (external motivators) for change are not usually as successful as personal motivations (internal). In the UK and in other countries around the world it is unlikely that financial incentives would or could be offered. However all health and social care providers are interested in **cost effectiveness.** Using the best, most effective or most acceptable therapy or intervention is likely to be best value. There is also the potential financial costs that come with **litigation** or complaints arising from mistakes or errors made when practitioners do not use the best available evidence.

Leaving behind the possibilities of financial benefit, many learning and change theorists, for example Knowles *et al.* (2005) have explored the importance of adult learning and how different things motivate different learners. Knowles *et al.* (2005) argue that adults learn more when they are involved and active, when their prior experience is recognized and their motivations explored. Generally people are more likely to change their behaviour if there are perceived rewards rather than punishments. However it is a complex process; Greenhalgh (2010: 204) says that there is no 'magic bullet' and there is unlikely to be in the future.

The power of people

Although there is no overall agreement of what strategies might help to get evidence in practice, there are many small studies that outline how various people in various roles impact on the implementation of evidence based practice in their own particular context. Some are profession or speciality specific.

See if you can find any primary research on the specific implementation of evidence in your own profession or speciality

The influence of those in executive roles

Having someone in a senior position within the organization to promote EBP can influence its use (Gifford *et al.* 2007; Sredl 2011). Here is a small sample of studies that have identified this:

Sredl *et al.* (2011) carried out a survey of nurse executives in the USA and found that although these leaders were supportive of EBP their actual implementation was relatively low. They concluded (p. 78) that *'executives must be the change agents'* who nurture the environment. Melynk and Davison (2009) add they should model EBP and create a culture of its acceptance.

Wilkinson *et al.* (2011) adopted a case study approach (using observation, documentary evidence and interviews) to explore **managers' potential to take on the role of facilitating** EBP. They found that managers were passively involved in EBP and that they prioritized managerial and administrative duties above those to facilitate EBP. They also recognized the complexity of the implementation of EBP and questioned who may best facilitate its implementation. If however, the individual is skilled and knowledgeable, they found that this can be successful.

In a mixed method study, Ploeg *et al.* (2010) reported that **'Best practice champions'** can influence the use of best practice guidelines through disseminating information, being persuasive and adapting guidelines to the **context** they are in.

In a Cochrane Review, Flodgren *et al.* (2010) tentatively found that **opinion leaders** may promote EBP. Their results are based on a wide range of studies with varied interventions and settings.

There is some evidence – though by no means extensive – that having a senior member of staff in support of EBP will facilitate its development.

Experts and specialists

Experts and specialists may also be influential in leading and developing an evidence-based approach within an organization. Experts and specialists may be accessible through personal contacts, networking and specialist interest groups in addition to their professional role. Such experts such as **specialists** in a particular field may have access to colleagues who may be able to reach agreed decisions on what is best practice. There are many published 'consensus statements'. Such papers can capture knowledge and skills that come from a vast range of practical experience in the field, for example Gray *et al.* (2011) provide a consensus guidance for use of wound debridement techniques in the UK. Do ensure you appraise their validity and expertise.

Here are some **examples** of the studies that have identified the positive role of experts and specialists:

Gerrish *et al.* (2011) presents a **case study** of 23 advanced practice nurses (APNs) from hospital and primary care settings across seven Strategic Health Authorities in England. She found that APNs promoted EBP among clinical nurses. They generated different types of evidence, accumulated evidence for clinical nurses, synthesized different forms of evidence, translated evidence by evaluating, interpreting and distilling it and disseminated evidence in a variety of ways.

Dogherty *et al.* (2010: 76) explored the facilitation skills of experts, describing the role as 'supporting and enabling practitioners to improve practice through evidence implementation'.

It is encouraging that new and emerging expert and specialist roles may provide a platform for practitioners to have real influence on decision making. Such roles include consultant roles, specialist practitioners, specialists or leads in education and professional development. Leaders should consider how such roles may be best used within their organizations. However there is one important (if obvious) point to be made: **learning from experts (role modelling) only works well if the role model is drawing on current evidence-based information and research to inform their practice.** Clearly, if we role model unsafe or out-of-date practices then ritualistic practice thrives (as discussed in Chapter 2). If practitioners are not up to date, this is likely to have a big influence on colleague and student learning. There is the potential for practice to be based on ritual rather than evidence if both students and practitioners fail to be open to challenge in their practice.

Evaluation of successful strategies for the implementation of EBP

It seems logical that shared understanding or culture can positively impact on the implementation and effectiveness of EBP and there is some evidence that those in senior positions within an organization and those in expert or specialist roles can influence the development of an evidence-based approach. Given the importance of developing an evidence-based culture, many observers, **for example** Melnyk *et al.* (2010) are keen to emphasize that it is essential to get strong evidence about the impact of EBP in the context of real practice.

Despite the evidence from the smaller studies mentioned previously, there is an absence of evidence about the overall impact on patient and client care when the organization adopts an evidence-based approach. Parmelli *et al.* (2011) reviewed the effectiveness of strategies to change organizational culture to improve healthcare performance. They give a full overview of the state of evidence in this area and conclude that at present, there is no clear evidence. Foxcroft and Cole (2009), and Flodgren *et al.* (2012), also undertook systematic reviews and found no clear evidence of an effect of the organizational approach to EBP or the effect on patient or client care.

In other studies, McGowan *et al.* (2009) explored the effectiveness of interventions that provided increased access to information and improvements in practice and patient care. Their review was also inconclusive due to a lack of good quality studies. Horsley *et al.* (2011) reviewed the teaching of critical appraisal skills in healthcare settings. Whilst they found some evidence that some critical appraisal teaching interventions may result in modest gains, again, the research question could not be fully answered due to lack of evidence.

It is important to note that **lack of evidence** does not mean that these organizational approaches don't work, it is just that we don't yet have the evidence and that further research is needed.

Finding solutions to the problems of implementing EBP

We have looked at the individual and organizational barriers to implementing EBP. Given that, even at organizational level, attitudes and approaches to EBP are influenced by individuals, it is possible to conclude that it is the individual who is critical in promoting an evidence-based approach. Referring back to the top **10 barriers to implementing evidence based practice** by Kajermo *et al.* (2010) we have developed the following strategies that can be adopted by individuals at every level within an organization to promote an evidence-based approach.

Strategy 1: Develop your own knowledge and skills

Throughout this book we have given you a *'Beginner's guide to evidence-based practice'*. We have explored how to search for high-quality evidence; if you are a student, your course will undoubtedly cover this in detail – do make the most of the practice and library sessions you are allocated.

If you are a qualified practitioner, seek out opportunities to learn how to search for evidence and ask your students to help you if you remain unsure. It is good practice for them and you!

We have addressed how to critically appraise the research and to help with this we have offered specific and general appraisal tools and checklists. We recommend that initially you could use our **'Six Questions to Trigger Critical Thinking'** (Aveyard *et al.* 2011) when you hear, see or read something that relates to your practice. Although we have not covered statistics in depth – many researchers use statisticians to help them – we have provided several glossaries and helpful websites that can help you understand statistical findings. You should also read the discussion part of research or if it is a systematic review, see if they have a summary of the paper to more easily explain their findings. Try and learn about some of the common phrases you read as you develop as an evidence-based practitioner.

As you become more skilled and knowledgeable you could access more advanced books and sources of information to further expand your knowledge and we would strongly recommend that you practise some of the skills – such as formulating a question, searching etc. in order to become proficient. We have emphasized the importance of systematic reviews and good literature reviews which summarize the available evidence on a topic. If a literature search fails to identify any reviews, consider whether you could undertake a review yourself with the help of your colleagues or if you are about to commence an academic course of study, consider whether you could undertake a review as a component of your course.

Part of being accountable for our practice is to recognize and address any limitations in our knowledge and skills and seek out further education.

Strategy 2: Increase your awareness of research

We have addressed this throughout this book. You may have never studied research methods or were not taught how to adopt a critical approach to literature – this sometimes depends on where or when you started your training. However nowadays, most health and social care practitioners are educated to a minimum of degree level and for most EBP is incorporated into their courses and competencies. So you could ask students to help you with this area whilst you share your expertise in professional practice.

If you supervise students then find out what evidence they are using in their course. They have access to up-to-date lectures, seminars and library resources and you may be able to learn from them.

Make the most of educational and development opportunities offered within your working day. Attend journal clubs and seminars on offer even if you do not feel that you will offer a big contribution. You will soon realise that you have some useful contributions to make. Melnyk *et al.* (2010) note that there are a variety of ways to successfully share EBP initiatives such as: practice rounds, presentations at conferences, and reports in journals, newsletters, and wider publications.

Brown *et al.* (2008) in their questionnaire study found that respondents had individual visions of what would facilitate research awareness and utilization. These ideas included:

- Emphasis on a team approach to problem solving
- Research shared at staff meetings
- Updates in a newsletter
- Research posters

> **Example:** Sortedahl (2012) organized online journal clubs in three different settings. They found that knowledge of EBP was increased in those who were involved in the journal clubs and that they shared evidence and developed contacts with each other and the researchers.

Strategy 3: Use summaries or syntheses of evidence

For busy practitioners it is important be able to be focussed in how we use our time. As part of our working day, we are unlikely to be able to stop what we are doing and carry out a literature search! Therefore, we need to be aware of how we can access information that has already been summarized or synthesized for us.

There is a move worldwide to provide 'synthesized evidence' which is made easily available to practitioners. These can be in a variety of forms such as: **evidence-based . . .**

- Websites offering access to systematic reviews and knowledge summaries
- Guidelines
- Policy
- Care pathways.

There is recognition that providing synthesized summaries of evidence that are accessible to busy practitioners may be a better way of getting evidence into practice.

We have discussed using specific databases in detail in Chapter 5 but here and in the useful web links at the back of this book, we offer some broader resources that offer collections of evidence.

As a starting point for finding the best available evidence:

Cochrane's 'webliography' of evidenced-based practice resources – it is an overview of the most important print and online resources for evidence-based healthcare and medicine (http://www.cochrane.org/about-us/evidence-based-health-care/webliography).

Evidence in Health and Social Care is another very good site that offers further links to a variety of resources. It aims to help people from across the NHS, public health and social care sectors to make better decisions as a result (http://www.evidence.nhs.uk/). There is a specific **public health** section (http://www.evidence.nhs.uk/nhs-evidence-content/public-health).

Try accessing a few of the websites offered at the back of this book and see which ones you find useful for your particular profession and speciality.

Using guidelines, policy and care pathways

Rotter *et al.* (2010) undertook a review to explore the effects of use of clinical pathways on professional practice. A **care pathway** is defined (p.1) as a 'structured multidisciplinary care plan used by health services to detail essential steps in the care of patients with a specific problem'. Overall, they found that use of pathways led to reduced length of stay, reduced in-hospital complications and improved documentation. Remind yourself, by reading Chapter 4, about using evidence-based guidelines and policy as a more accessible form of evidence for your practice.

Remember to critically appraise guidelines as explored in Chapter 6 as they may not be evidence based or up to date.

Strategy 4: Make the most of your time

Being under-staffed, too busy to think and unable to get all our work done have been constant issues in most health and social care workers' lives. Time management is widely discussed in the literature and strategies are offered to help us manage our time better. It is therefore worth thinking about ways and means of incorporating evidence in our practice in a more time effective way. Guides to help us prioritize sometimes offer the idea that we should consider what is **URGENT** and what is **IMPORTANT** when making priority decisions. Also in this chapter we offer some resources that can help save time such as systematic reviews, guidelines, care pathways and synthesized knowledge summaries. Consider the time that will be saved if there is a **clear and consistent approach** to care that will result in the best outcomes for your patients/clients.

Time is our most precious resource and busy practitioners 'keep their heads down' and do what they need to do to get the job done. Evidence-based practice seems to be an optional extra. This then becomes a wider organizational issue where strong leadership has potential to influence change. Managers should ensure that **staffing levels should incorporate time for developing and implementing an evidence-based approach** to practice. This then shows that professional development is valued within the organization.

Try considering the following:

- Do what you can to incorporate EBP as part of your role or daily work rather than as an add-on.
- Be prepared for when there are slacker periods to 'find/read evidence', i.e. keep articles, guidelines and other evidence available and ready to read when you have some spare time.
- See if you can network with others in similar specialities so that you can combine your efforts.
- Develop a questioning culture so you can share information with colleagues.
- Agree that you will ask each other why you approach a task or intervention in a particular way and try and find out if there is any evidence for that approach.
- Ask any students you have on placement to talk about what they are learning in university (ask them to bring in relevant articles/lecture notes or even do a presentation to the team).
- See if your student has time/need to investigate a specific issue and see if they would be interested in doing a literature review on a topic relevant to your practice.
- Ask experts/specialists for any summaries/guidelines they know of relating to your speciality (remember to critically appraise them).
- Start by accessing sites that contain systematic reviews or knowledge summaries or EBP journals rather than individual articles or books.
- Take turns in finding out the best available evidence on a topic and present it at team meetings.
- Ensure any staff member who attends a study day/conference or course feeds back to the wider team any implications for practice.
- Try and build in the evidence base for your other priorities (targets, projects or strategies) and see how it relates to improving patient/client outcomes.

- Consider if attending a clinical/professional conference or doing a course would be a faster/more effective way of ensuring your practice is up to date.

Strategy 5: Develop authority and confidence to influence and obtain resources and support

Some of these areas may be outside your control, but think about what you can do. Consider if you have communicated any resource/support needs in a constructive and assertive way. Talk to colleagues and see if they feel the same and find someone with influence who can act on your behalf. Your own confidence will develop as you become more knowledgeable about research and EBP.

We have discussed how leadership may impact on the adoption of EBP. But if the leader in your workplace is unsupportive you may have to develop wider support from networking and from colleagues further afield such as experts. Ask yourself why some colleagues may be unsupportive of EBP; it may be because they are under pressure themselves, are threatened by change or may not see what you want to do as a priority. Communication is the key! Ask them what their reasons are and try to explore a solution together – compromise is often the answer.

Challenging the practice of ourselves and others

As we discussed throughout earlier in this book it is hard to move from practices that we are familiar and comfortable with. We have discussed how the individual as well as the organization can influence the update of EBP. One of the reasons why both students and qualified practitioners are reluctant to bring in new ideas is a **fear of challenging what has always been done.** We often hear from our students that they try and share with their practice assessors/mentors things they have learnt but are met with a defensive or reluctant response rather than an open and interested attitude.

Think about how you and your team react to having your practice challenged. Is it seen as a way of professionally developing or as a personal criticism? Could you do more to invite challenge to your practice – give permission for others to question you?

Most people would welcome feedback to improve their practice, although it is worth recognizing that in a busy working environment or if practice is challenged in an untactful way then our natural reaction would be to be defensive.

This is more likely if practice is challenged in an accusatory way; there are more subtle ways that practice can be challenged which might prevent a 'defensive response'.

Remember you are accountable for your own practice and you may have to be assertive.

> **Example:** it is easier to put forward a suggestion for a change in practice if you are sure about the evidence underpinning your assertion and can produce the source of that evidence.

 Think of a time when someone has challenged you about something that was entirely justifiable. If they approached you in a tactful way you were probably more likely to accept what they were saying than if they confronted you directly.

Ideas for adopting a more open approach to challenging practice

- Discuss in advance with colleagues/practice educators/students what you should do if you see practice that conflicts with evidence you are aware of.
- Before you challenge the practice of others, consider the validity of the evidence you have – *might there be things you are unaware of, for example, context, more than one approach or different values?*
- Try and start a conversation with someone where you ask them tactfully about the evidence underpinning their decision.
  - Ask for their perspective on the issue/your observations.
  - Offer to share that you have just found a new way of doing something.
  - Ask if you can help to find the evidence for a particular therapy or intervention.
  - Consider asking questions rather than making accusations about practice.
  - Give them time to consider your view or question.
  - Suggest the issue as a topic for a journal club or team project.
- Consider if the practice is unsafe or inappropriate; your role might be as an advocate for your patients or clients – this may help you to be assertive.
- Consider the setting; avoid challenging another practitioner in public unless the practice is unsafe. Ask to speak to them privately.

 Consider now what you would do if you spotted unsafe or out-of-date practice by a colleague, practice educator or student.

> At Oxford Brookes University, we have produced **guidelines for students regarding how to manage concerns in practice placements** (http://www.hls. brookes.ac.uk/images/pdfs/plu/plc05a_guidelines-for-raising-and-escalating-concerns.pdf).
>
> **NHS employers** have a series of resources and materials that organizations can display, they also have links to other **professional bodies'** guides and advice. (http://www.nhsemployers.org/employmentpolicyandpractice/ukemployment-practice/raisingconcerns/pages/whistleblowing.aspx).

Adopting some of these approaches may help you in moving from ritualistic or routine approaches to professional practice to a more evidence-based approach.

The future of evidence-based practice

There are a variety of views being debated in the literature regarding the value of EBP and its place as part of a wider spectrum of the art, values and science of professional health and social care. These sometimes diverse but often overlapping views are a valuable part of a healthy debate ensuring the focus for practitioners is on delivery of a safe, effective and compassionate health and social care. There is undoubtedly more work to do in the education of practitioners to develop the knowledge, skills and positive attitudes to searching and appraising evidence so it can be used alongside clinical/professional judgement and patient/client preferences in their decision making.

Increasingly there is emphasis on overcoming barriers and finding a range of ways to successfully implement evidence into practice and evaluate these approaches and the positive outcomes for patients/clients. Although there is widespread reporting of context-specific examples, there is clearly need for more, high-quality and wider-reaching research.

In summary

Throughout this book we have identified that developing an EBP approach is both a personal and an organizational responsibility. As an individual, it is vital that you understand why EBP is an important aspect of delivering high standards of practice. All practitioners need to be aware of the need for EBP and to have the skills to search for, evaluate and understand the evidence they find. Then you need to be working within an organizational culture that is open and receptive to change and prepared to embrace the concept of using evidence in practice. Although the second stage is dependent on the culture of the organization, the culture of the organization is dependent on the individuals within it. There is increased recognition of the value of synthesized resources to help individual practitioners and organizations. There is much that you as an individual alongside your colleagues can do to support the development of this culture as outlined within this chapter.

We hope that you have found this introduction to EBP useful and relevant to your professional lives.

Key points

1 Developing EBP requires the practitioner to have the skills of finding and evaluating evidence.
2 This requires the motivation and dedication of the individual practitioner to achieve this.
3 Developing an EBP approach also requires an open organizational culture of accepting change and a supportive infrastructure.
4 Do not underestimate your individual contribution to this organizational culture as an individual – even as a student. Remember that the organization is made up of individuals.
5 There is increasing recognition that synthesized evidence such as in systematic reviews, policy and guidelines can help busy practitioners but more research is clearly needed.

Glossary

Abstract: A summary of a research or discussion paper. The abstract will give you a general overview of the paper but you are advised to access the whole paper if the paper is of interest to you.

Action research: A study carried out in a practical setting, often involving those working there. The results are implemented and evaluated within that setting.

Bias: Flaws in the design of a study that can lead to invalid conclusions.

Blinding: An approach used when either the participants or researchers (or both; double blind) are unaware of the full details of the study. Blinding is used to reduce bias in a study when awareness of some aspect of the study would be likely to affect behaviour.

Campbell Collaboration: A worldwide collaboration who commission and maintain systematic reviews in social care.

Case control study: A study in which people with a specific condition (cases) are compared to people without this condition (controls) to compare the frequency of the occurrence of the exposure that might have caused the disease.

Clinical practice guideline: A summary of current evidence to assist professionals make decisions about care.

Clinical trial: A study undertaken in a clinical area to compare the effect of an intervention. The term clinical trial often refers to a Randomized Controlled Trial.

Cochrane Collaboration: A worldwide collaboration who commission and maintain systematic reviews in healthcare.

Coding: The process of giving a code to a piece of qualitative data in order to help with analysis. Codes are then combined into categories for further analysis.

Cohort study: A study in which two or more groups or cohorts are followed up to examine whether exposures measured at the beginning lead to outcomes, such as disease.

Confidence interval: Confidence intervals are usually (but arbitrarily) 95 per cent confidence intervals. A reasonable, though strictly incorrect interpretation, is that the 95 per cent confidence interval gives the range in which the population effect lies. A wide confidence interval implies a lack of certainty or precision about the true population effect and is commonly found in studies with too few participants.

Confirmability: In qualitative research, this refers to the extent to which the results can be confirmed. This sometimes leads to asking participants to verify the statements made in the interview, but not all researchers ascribe to this view.

Confounding factors: Other factors that influence the results of a study – these can generally be eliminated by randomization.

CONSORT statement: A statement that describes the information that should be included in the report of a trial.

Convenience sample: A sample that is obtained due to convenience factors – for example, all those attending a seminar are invited to fill in a questionnaire.

Credibility: Evidence from the study that the results or conclusions are believable. This term is often used in the evaluation of qualitative studies.

Critical appraisal: A process by which the quality of evidence is assessed, evaluated or questioned, often using a critical appraisal tool.

Critical appraisal tool: A list of questions or checklist used to help assess the quality of evidence.

Database: A collection of data; in research, a database normally refers to a collection of journals that are searchable electronically.

Dependability: This term is often used in qualitative research to describe the extent to which the researcher can account for the methods and results found in the study.

Descriptive statistics: Statistics such as means, medians, standard deviations, that describe aspects of the data, such as central tendency (mean or median) or its dispersion (standard deviation).

Discourse analysis: An approach to analyse the use of language in order to understand meaning in complex areas.

Discussion paper: A paper presenting an argument or discussion that does not contain empirical research findings.

Dissertation: A document presenting the method and the main findings from a piece of academic work.

Double blind study: A study in which neither the researchers nor the participants are aware of which treatment or intervention the participants are receiving.

Effect size: The size of the effect; the difference between the intervention and the control group in an experiment.

Empirical research: Research which is carried out in the 'field' where data is collected first hand. It is often based on observation or experiment and written up as a research study.

Essay: A short piece of academic writing on a selected topic. An essay might contain reference to research but is not a research study.

Ethnography: Qualitative research approach which involves the study of culture/way of life of participants.

Evidence-based practice: Practice which is based on the best available evidence, moderated by patient preferences and clinical/professional judgement.

Exclusion criteria: Criteria that are set in order to focus the searching strategy for a literature review (e.g. not children, not acute care episodes).

Experimental research: A study designed to test whether a treatment or intervention is effective.

Forest plot: A graph which illustrates the spread of individual results combined in a meta-analysis. The plot displays the extent to which all the studies in a review have similar or dissimilar results.

Generalize: To apply the findings of one study to the wider population. Generalizability refers to quantitative research only as qualitative studies do not seek to generalize (see definition of transferability below). Remember you cannot generalize from anecdotal evidence.

Gold standard: A procedure or method which is widely regarded as being the best available.

Grounded theory: Qualitative research approach that involves exploration of a topic about which little is known and results in the generation of theory.

Guideline: A systematically developed statement to assist practitioners in the delivery of evidence-based care.

Hierarchy of evidence: A grading system for ranking the best form of evidence to answer a specific question. Remember there is no one hierarchy of evidence – it all depends on the question!

Inclusion (and exclusion) criteria: Criteria that are set in order to focus the searching strategy for a literature review (e.g. research from the past five years, published in English).

Inferential statistics: Statistics that are used to apply findings from the sample population to the wider population, usually meaning statistical tests.

Intervention: An activity which is intended to improve or effect health or social care outcomes.

Journal: An academic publication in which researchers publish their research. There are academic journals for many subjects and disciplines.

Key terms: Terms used when searching for literature using an electronic database that represents the focus of the topic you need to study. Academic papers entered into the database are indexed using key terms.

Limitations: A statement in a research paper (or literature review) which refers to what could be criticized about the research process undertaken and which subsequently affects the validity of the results.

Literature review: A collection of research papers and other evidence on a particular topic. A good literature (or systematic review) should let you know precisely how they carried out the review.

MeSH: Medical Subject Headings: a thesaurus of medical terms used to index medical information in some databases.

Meta-analysis: A process by which quantitative data (with similar properties) is combined to produce a weighted average of all the results.

Meta-ethnography: A process by which the results of qualitative data are combined.

Meta-study: A process by which the results of qualitative data are combined.

Mind map: A graph or chart that helps to make sense of random thoughts or thoughts from a brainstorm.

Narrative review: An approach to undertaking a literature review, but not one that is undertaken according to a predefined or systematic approach.

Non-empirical evidence: Evidence that is not based on the findings of research.

Odds ratio: The odds of an event occurring in the experimental group, divided by the odds of an event occurring in the control group.

Outcome: The end result or consequence (of a study). The outcome is often the focal point of a study.

P.I.C.O.T: Acronym whose initials represent Population, Intervention/Issue Comparsion/Context, Outcome and Time – sometimes shortened to **PICO**.

Peer review: The process in which experts in a subject area are invited to review the academic work of an author, often prior to publication in a journal.

Phenomenology: Qualitative research approach in which the participants' 'lived experience' is explored.

Primary research/research study: A study undertaken using a planned and methodological approach.

Professional judgement: Considered judgement made by a professional when making a decision. Professional judgement is a component of evidence-based practice.

Purposive sampling: Sampling strategy used by qualitative researchers who are looking for a population that is 'fit for the purposes' of the study in question.

P values: p for probability. The p value is the probability of observing results or results more extreme than those observed if the null hypothesis was true.

Qualitative research: Research that involves an in-depth understanding of the reasons for and meanings of human behaviour – the results are often presented in words.

Quantitative research: Research that involves collecting data that can be defined in categories and presented numerically.

Questionnaire: A list of questions to be asked of respondents, sometimes called a survey.

Randomization: The process of allocating individuals randomly to groups, usually in a Randomized Controlled Trial to ensure that two or more groups in a trial are equal in terms of participants' characteristics.

Randomized controlled trial: A trial which has randomly assigned groups in order to determine the effectiveness of an intervention(s) which is given to one/two other of the groups.

Random sampling: A sampling strategy in which everyone in a given population has an equal chance of being selected and that probability is independent of any other person selected.

Relevance: Research that can be applied to my patient or client group and context. This term is often used in the evaluation of qualitative studies.

Reliability: The extent to which the same result in a study will be repeated if the same methods are used. This term is generally applied to quantitative research methods.

Reproducibility: The extent to which the study, or parts of the study, could be repeated in other settings by other people.

Research methodology: The process undertaken in order to address the research question – for example, Randomized Controlled Trial, ethnographic study and so on.

Research question: A question set by researchers at the outset of a study, to be addressed in the study. See PICOT.

Research study/primary study: A study undertaken using a planned and methodological approach including a research question, method of obtaining data and results and conclusions.

Reviews of research: A collection of research on a particular topic. If the review is not referred to as systematic, check to see if the method of undertaking the search is clearly defined – if it is not it is likely to be less reliable.

Rigour: The term applied to the assessment of the way in which a study has been undertaken. A rigorous study is one that has been carried out meticulously. A study that lacks rigour is one that is haphazard in design.

Risk ratio: The ratio of risk of an event occurring in the experimental group divided by the risk in the control group.

Sample: The group of people included in a study. This can be a random or convenience sample for a quantitative study, or a purposive or theoretical sample for a qualitative study.

Search strategy: A planned strategy for searching the literature. A comprehensive search strategy is a component of undertaking a rigorous review.

Secondary source: A source which the reader has not accessed themselves – but has used someone else's representation or interpretation of it.

Snowball sampling: A sampling strategy in which who/what is involved in the study (sample) is determined according to the needs of the study as the investigation progresses.

Standard deviation: Shows the variation or deviation from the mean or average.

Statistical significance: The level of significance (p value) is the probability of having observed the data in a study when the null hypothesis is true.

Statistics: Statistics is the collection, organization and analysis of numerical data. Statistics are generally used in quantitative studies to represent the data collected. Two different types of statistics are commonly used in quantitative research; descriptive and inferential statistics (defined above).

Stratification: The sample is divided into groups that have the same value, for example, stratifying by age means putting people of the same age or age group together.

Strengths: In the context of evidence-based practice, strengths refer to the positive points in a study which give the evidence more weight.

Systematic review: A very detailed review of the literature that is undertaken according to a defined and systematic approach. The way in which the review was carried out will be clearly detailed.

Theoretical sampling: An approach to sampling in grounded theory where the sampling strategy evolves as the study progresses, according to the needs of the study and the developing theory.

Transferability: Transferability refers to the extent to which the results or findings of a study may be transferred to (or have meaning for) another context or population. Transferability is usually used in qualitative research where the aim is not to generalize, but to consider the extent to which significant concepts identified may be transferable to other contexts.

Trustworthiness: Trustworthiness refers to the honest and reliable reporting of a study. This term is often related only to qualitative studies.

Validity: the extent to which a study or an intervention measures what it is intended to measure.

References

Allen, N.E., Beral V., Casabonne, D., Sau Wan Kan, Reeves, G.K., Brown A. and Green J. (2009) Moderate alcohol intake and cancer incidence in women. *Journal of the National Cancer Institute* 101(5): 296–305

Aveyard, H. (2010) *Doing a Literature Review in Health and Social Care* 2nd edn. Open University Press: Maidenhead

Aveyard, H., Sharp, P. and Woolliams, M. (2011) *A Beginner's Guide to Critical Thinking and Writing in Health and Social Care*. Open University Press: Maidenhead

Benner, P. (1984) *From Novice to Expert*. Addison Wesley Publishing Company: New York

Benner, P. and Tanner, C.A. (1987) Clinical judgement: how expert nurses use intuition *American Journal of Nursing* 87(1): 23–31

Birnbaum, R. and Saini, M. (2012) Synthesis of children's participation in custody disputes. *Research on Social Work Practice* 22: 400–409, doi:10.1177/1049731512442985

Bradshaw, A. and Price, L. (2006) Rectal suppositories insertion: the reliability of the evidence as a basis for nursing practice. *Journal of Clinical Nursing* 16(1): 98–103

Brady, M.C., Kinn, S., Ness, V., O'Rourke, K., Randhawa, N. and Stuart, P. (2009) Preoperative fasting for preventing perioperative complications in children. *Cochrane Database of Systematic Reviews Issue* 4. Art. No.: CD005285. DOI: 10.1002/14651858.CD005285.pub2

Brown, C.E., Wickline, M.A., Ecoff L. and Galser, D. (2008) Nursing practice, knowledge, attitudes and perceived barriers to evidence based practice at an academic medical centre. *Journal of Advanced Nursing* 65(2): 371–381

Burls, A. (2009) *What is Critical Appraisal?* 2nd edn. Haywood Medical Communications: Newmarket UK available at http://www.medicine.ox.ac.uk/bandolier/painres/download/whatis/what_is_critical_appraisal.pdf

CASP International Network (2010) available at www.caspinternational.org

Crabtree, J.L., Justiss, M. and Swinehart, S. (2012) Occupational therapy masters-level students' evidence-based practice knowledge and skills before and after fieldwork. *Occupational Therapy in Health Care*, 26(92–3): 138–149

CONSORT (2010) the CONSORT statement available at http://www.consort-statement.org.

Cottrell, S. (2011) *Critical Thinking Skills* 2nd edn. Palgrave MacMillan: Basingstoke

Crowe, M. and Sheppard, I. (2011) A review of critical appraisal tools show they lack rigor: alternative tool structure is proposed. *Journal of Clinical Epidemiology* 64(1):79–89

Crowe, M., Sheppard, L. and Campbell, A. (2012) Reliability analysis for a proposed critical appraisal tool demonstrated value for diverse research designs. *Journal of Clinical Epidemiology* 65: 375e–383

Dawes, M., Summerskill, W. and Glasziou, P. *et al.* (2005) Sicily statement on evidence-based practice. *BMC Medical Education* 5(1): 1–7 available at http://www.biomedcentral.com/1472-6920/5/1

Department of Constitutional Affairs (2005) *Mental Capacity Act: Code Of Practice.* The Stationery Office: London

Department of Health (DH 2010) *Essence of Care.* DH: London available at: http://www.dh.gov.uk/en/Publicationsandstatistics/Publications/PublicationsPolicy-AndGuidance/DH_119969

Department of Health (DH 2012) *Liberating the NHS – No Decision About Me Without Me* consultation document DH: London http://www.dh.gov.uk/en/Consultations/Liveconsultations/DH_134221

Dixon-Woods, M., Sutton, A., Shaw, R., Miller, T., Smith, J., Young, B., Bonas, S., Booth, A. and Jones, D. (2007) Appraising qualitative research for inclusion in systematic reviews: a quantitative and qualitative comparison of three methods. *Journal of Health Service Research Policy* 12(1): 42–47

Dogherty, E.J., Harrison, M.B. and Graham, I.D. (2010) Facilitation as a role and process in achieving evidence-based practice in nursing: a focused review of concept and meaning. *Worldviews on Evidence-Based Nursing* 7(2): 76–89

Doll, R. and Hill, A.B. (1954) The mortality of doctors in relation to their smoking habits, *British Medical Journal* 228: 1451–1455

Downie, R. and Macnaughton, J. (2009) In defence of professional judgement. *Advances in Psychiatric Treatment* 15(5): 322–327

Eckmanns, T., Bessert, J., Behnke, M., Gastmeier, P. and Ruden, H. (2006) Compliance with antiseptic hand rub use in intensive care units: the Hawthorne effect. *Infection Control and Hospital Epidemiology* 27(9): 931–934

Elliott, N. (2003) Portfolio creation, action research and the learning environment: a study from probation. *Qualitative Social Work* 2(3): 327–345

Ericsson, I., Hellstrom, I. and Kjellstrom, S. (2011) Sliding interactions: an ethnography about how persons with dementia interact in housing with care for the elderly. *Dementia* 4(10): 523–538

Ernst, E. (2008) Treating the evidence with contempt (letter). *British Medical Journal* 337:a2063 doi: 10.1136/bmj.a2063

Farley, A.C., Hajek, P., Lycett, D. and Aveyard, P. (2012) Interventions for preventing weight gain after smoking cessation. *Cochrane Database of Systematic Reviews* http://onlinelibrary.wiley.com/doi/10.1002/14651858.CD006219.pub3/abstract

Fineout-Overholt, E. and Johnston, L. (2005) Teaching evidence based practice: asking searchable, answerable clinical questions. *World Views on Evidence-based Nursing* 2(3): 157–160

Fineout-Overholt, E., Melnyk, B.M. Stillwell, S. and Williamson, K.M. (2010) Evidence-based practice: step by step: critical appraisal of the evidence: Part I. *American Journal of Nursing:* 110(7): 47–52

Fisher, J. and Clayton, M. (2012) Who gives a tweet: assessing patients' interest in the use of social media for health care. *Worldviews on Evidence-Based Nursing* 9(2): 100–108

Flodgren, G., Parmelli, E., Doumit, G., Gattellari, M., O'Brien, M.A., Grimshaw, J. and Eccles, M.P. (2010) Local opinion leaders: effects on professional practice and health care outcomes. *Cochrane Database of Systematic Reviews* available at http://onlinelibrary.wiley.com/doi/10.1002/14651858.CD000125.pub3/pdf

Flodgren, G., Rojas-Reyes, M.X., Cole, N. and Foxcroft, D.R. (2012) Effectiveness of organisational infrastructures to promote evidence-based nursing practice (Review) *Cochrane Database of Systematic Reviews* available at http://onlinelibrary.wiley.com/doi/10.1002/14651858.CD002212.pub2/pdf/standard

Foxcroft, D.R. and Cole, N. (2009) Organisational infrastructures to promote evidence based nursing practice. *Cochrane Database of Systematic Reviews* available at http://onlinelibrary.wiley.com/doi/10.1002/14651858.CD002212/pdf/standard

Fraser, A.G. and Dunstan, F.D. (2010) On the impossibility of being expert. *British Medical Journal* 341 doi: 10.1136/bmj.c6815

Fullford, K.W.M. (2010) Bringing together values-based and evidence-based medicine: UK Department of Health Initiatives in the `Personalization' of Care. *Journal of Evaluation in Clinical Practice* 17(2): 341–343

Furlong, M., McGilloway, S., Bywater, T., Hutchings, J., Smith, S.M. and Donnelly, M. (2012) Behavioural and cognitive-behavioural group-based parenting programmes for early-onset conduct problems in children aged 3 to 12 years. *Cochrane Database of Systematic Reviews* 2. Available at http://onlinelibrary.wiley.com/doi/10.1002/14651858.CD008225.pub2/pdf

Gardner, A.W., Parker, D.E., Montgomery, P.S., Scott, K.J. and Blevins, S.M. (2011) Efficacy of quantified home-based exercise and supervised exercise in patients with intermittent claudication; a randomized controlled trial. *Circulation* 123: 491–498

Gerrish, K., McDonnell, A.M., Nolan, M., Guillaume, L., Kirshbaum, M. and Tod, A. (2011) The role of advanced practice nurses in knowledge brokering as a means of promoting evidence-based practice among clinical nurses. *Journal of Advanced Nursing* 67(9): 2004–2014

Gifford, W., Davies, B., Edwards, N., Griffin, P. and Lybanon, V. (2007) Managerial leadership for nurses' use of research evidence: an integrative review of the literature. *Worldviews on Evidence-Based Nursing* 4: 126–145. doi: 10.1111/j.1741-6787.2007.00095.x

Gilson, L., Hanson, K., Sheikh, K., Agyepong, I.A., Ssengooba, F. and Bennett, S. (2011) Building the field of health policy and systems research: social science matters. *PLoS medicine* 8 (8) http://resyst.lshtm.ac.uk/sites/resyst.lshtm.ac.uk/files/docs/reseources/PLOS_2.pdf

Goldacre, B. (2008) *Bad Science*. Harper Collins: London

Gray, D., Acton, C., Chadwick, P., Fumarola, S., Leaper, D., Morris, C., Stang, D., Vowden, K., Vowden, P. and Young, T. (2011) Consensus guidance for the use of debridement techniques in the UK. *Wounds UK*, 7(1): 77–84

Greenhalgh, T. (2010) *How to Read a Paper: The Basics of Evidence-based Medicine*. John Wiley: Oxford

Greenhalgh, T. and Peacock, R. (2005) Effectiveness and efficiency of search methods in systematic reviews of complex evidence: audit of primary sources. *British Medical Journal* 331: 1064–1065

Hastie, R. and Dawes, R.M. (2010) *Rational Choice in an Uncertain World*, 2nd edn. Sage Publications: Thousand Oaks, California

Health and Care Professions Council (HCPC) (2012) *Standards of Conduct, Performance and Ethics* available at http=//www.hpc-uk.org/aboutregistration/standards/

Hodges, B.D. (2008) Discourse analysis. *British Medical Journal* 337: a879

Horsley, T., Hyde, C., Santesso, N., Parkes, J., Milne, R. and Stewart, R. (2011) Teaching critical appraisal skills in healthcare settings (Review). *Cochrane Database of Systematic Reviews* available at. http://onlinelibrary.wiley.com/doi/10.1002/14651858.CD001270.pub2/pdf/standard

Howe, W. (2001) Evaluating quality. Available at http://www.walthowe.com/navnet/quality.html

Jefferson, T., Del Mar, C.B., Dooley, L., Ferroni, E., Al-Ansary, L.A., Bawazeer, G.A., van Driel, M.L., Nair, S., Jones, M.A., Thorning, S. and Conly, J.M. (2011) Physical interventions to interrupt or reduce the spread of respiratory viruses. *Cochrane Database of Systematic Reviews* available at http://onlinelibrary.wiley. com/doi/10.1002/14651858.CD006207.pub4/abstract

Kajermo, K.N., Boström, A.M., Thompson, D.S., Hutchinson, A.M., Estabrooks, C.A. and Wallin, L. (2010) The BARRIERS scale – the barriers to research utilization scale: a systematic review. *Implementation Science* 5:(32): 1–22 available at http://www.implementationscience.com/content/5/1/32

Katrak, P., Blalocerkowski, A.E., Massy-Westropp, N., Saravana Kumar, V.S. and Grimmer, K.A. (2004) A systematic review of the content of critical appraisal tools. *BMC Medical Research Methodology* 2004 (4) 22: 1–11 http://www.biomed-central.com/content/pdf/1471-2288-4-22.pdf

Keenan, B., Atkins, C., Keenan, B., Jenkins, C., Denner, L., Harries, M., Fawcett, K., Atkins, S. and Miller, J. (2011) Promoting mental health in older people admitted to hospitals. *Nursing Standard* 25(20): 46–56

Kitson, A.L., Rycroft-Malone, J., Harvey, G., McCormack, B., Seers, K. and Titchen, A. (2008) Evaluating the successful implementation of evidence into practice using the PARiHS framework: theoretical and practical challenges. *Implementation Science* 3(1): 1–12 available at http://www.implementationscience.com/content/pdf/1748-5908-3-1.pdf

Kmietowicz, Z. (2012) University College London issues new research standards but says it won't investigate Wakefield *British Medical Journal* 345: e6220

Knipschild, P. (1994) Systematic Reviews – some examples. *British Medical Journal* 309:719–1

Knowles, M, Holton, E.F. and Swanson, R.A. (2005) *The Adult Learner: The Definitive Classic in Adult Education and Human Resource Development* 6th edn. Elsevier: Burlington, MA

Last, J.M. (ed.) (1988) *A Dictionary of Epidemiology.* Oxford University Press: New York

Lincoln, Y.S. and Guba, E.G. (1985) *Naturalistic Inquiry.* Sage Publications: Beverly Hills, CA

Manaseki-Holland, S., Bavuusuren, B., Bayandarj, T., Sprachman, S. and Marshall, T. (2010) Effects of traditional swaddling on development. a randomised controlled trial. *Paediatrics* 126(6): e1485 -e1492 doi: 10.1542/peds.2009-1531

Mangnall, J. and Yurkovich, E. (2010) A grounded theory exploration of deliberate self-harm in incarcerated women. *Journal of Forensic Nursing* 6(2): 88–95

McCluskey, A. and Bishop B (2009) The Adapted Fresno Test of competence in evidence-based practice. *Journal of Continuing Education in the Health Professions* 29(2):119–126

McGowan, J., Grad, R., Pluye, P., Hannes, K., Deane, K., Labrecque, M., Welch, V. and Tugwell, P. (2009) Electronic retrieval of health information by healthcare providers to improve practice and patient care. *Cochrane Database of Systematic Reviews* http://onlinelibrary.wiley.com/doi/10.1002/14651858.CD004749. pub2/abstract

McGraughey, J., Alderdice, F., Fowler, R., Kapila, A., Mayhew, A. and Moutray, M. (2009) Outreach and early warning systems for the prevention of intensive care admission and death of critically ill adult patients on general hospital wards (review). *Cochrane Database of Systematic Reviews* http://onlinelibrary.wiley.com/doi/10.1002/14651858.CD005529.pub2/abstract

Melnyk, B.M., Fineout-Overholt, E., Stillwell, B. and Williamson, K.M. (2009) Evidence-based practice: step by step: igniting a spirit of inquiry. *American Journal of Nursing* 109(11): 49–52

Melnyk, B.M. and Davison, S. (2009) Creating a culture of innovation in nursing education through shared vision, leadership, interdisciplinary partnerships, and positive deviance. *Nursing Administration Quarterly* 33(4): 288–295

Melnyk, B.M., Fineout-Overholt, E., Stillwell, S.B. and Williamson, K.M. (2010) Evidence-based practice: step by step: the seven steps of evidence-based practice. *American Journal of Nursing* 110(1): 51–53

Militello, L.K., Kelly, S.A. and Melnyk, B.M. (2012) Systematic review of text-messaging interventions to promote healthy behaviors in pediatric and adolescent populations: implications for clinical practice and research. *Worldviews on Evidence-Based Nursing* 9(2): 66–77

Nevo, I. and Slonim-Nevo, V. (2011) The Myth of evidence-based practice: towards evidence-informed practice. *British Journal of Social Work* 41(6): 1176–1197

Noyes, J. (2010) Never mind the qualitative feel the depth! The evolving role of qualitative research in Cochrane intervention reviews. *Journal of Research in Nursing* 15(6): 255–534

Nursing and Midwifery Council (NMC) (2008) *The Code: Standards of Conduct, Performance and Ethics for Nurses and Midwives*. NMC: London available at http://www.nmc-uk.org/Publications/Standards/

Nursing and Midwifery Council (NMC) (2010) *Essential Skills Clusters*. NMC: London available at http://standards.nmc-uk.org/Documents/Annexe3_%20ESCs_16092010.pdf

Oldershaw, M. (2009) *What are adult nursing students' attitudes towards patients with HIV/AIDS and what can be done to improve attitudes?* Unpublished BSc (hons) dissertation, School of Health and Social Care, Oxford Brookes University, Oxford

Parmelli, E., Flodgren, G., Schaafsma, M.E., Baillie, N., Beyer, F.R. and Eccles, M.P. (2011) The effectiveness of strategies to change organisational culture to improve healthcare performance (Review). *Cochrane Database of Systematic Reviews* available at http://onlinelibrary.wiley.com/doi/10.1002/14651858.CD008315.pub2/pdf/abstract

Pauling, L. (1986) *How to Live Longer and Feel Better*. Oregon State University Press: Oregon

Petter, J. and Armitage, E., (2012) Raising educational standards for the paramedic profession. *Journal of Paramedic Practice*, 4(4): 241–242

Ploeg, J., Skelly, J., Rowan, M., Edwards, N., Davies, B., Grinspun, D., Bajnok, I. and Downey, A. (2010) The role of nursing best practice champions in diffusing practice guidelines: a mixed methods study. *Worldviews on Evidence-Based Nursing* 7(4): 238–251

Price, B. and Harrington, A. (2010) *Critical Thinking and Writing for Nursing Students (transforming nursing practice)*. Learning Matters: Exeter

Rotter, T., Kinsman, L., James, E.L., Machotta, A., Gothe, H., Willis, J., Snow, P. and Kugler, J. (2010) Clinical pathways: effects on professional practice, patient outcomes, length of stay and hospital costs: *Cochrane Database of Systematic Reviews* Issue 3. Art. No.: CD006632. DOI: 10.1002/14651858.CD006632.pub2. available at http://onlinelibrary.wiley.com/doi/10.1002/14651858.CD006632.pub2/pdf/standard

Royal College of Nursing (RCN 2007) *Hospital hydration best practice toolkit.* Available at http://www.rcn.org.uk/newsevents/campaigns/nutritionnow/tools_and_resources/hydration

Sackett, D.L., Rosenberg, W.M.C., Muir Gray, J.A., Haynes, R.B. and Richardson, W.S. (1996) Evidence based medicine. What it is and what it isn't. *British Medical Journal* 312: 71–72

Sackett, D.L., Straus, S.E., Richardson, W.S., Rosenburg, W. and Haynes, R.B. (2000) *Evidence-based Medicine: How to Practise and Teach EBM.* London: Churchill Livingstone

Schofield, I., Tolson, D. and Fleming, V. (2011) How nurses understand and care for older people with delirium in the acute hospital: a Critical Discourse Analysis. *Nursing Inquiry* 19(2): 165–176

Schulz K.F., Altman, D.G. and Moher, D. (2011) CONSORT 2010 Statement: Updated Guidelines for Reporting Parallel Group Randomized Trials. *Annals of Internal Medicine* 152(11): 726–733

Sharp, P. and Taylor, B. (2012) *Prompt questions for Randomised Controlled Trials and qualitative studies* (unpublished). Oxford Brookes University: Oxford

Smith, R. (1991) Where is the wisdom . . .? the poverty of medical evidence. *British Medical Journal* 303: 798–799

Smith, R. (2010) Strategies for coping with information overload. *British Medical Journal* 341: c7126

Sortedahl, C. (2012) Effect of online journal club on evidence-based practice knowledge, intent, and utilization in school nurses. *Worldviews on Evidence-Based Nursing* 9(2): 117–125

Sredl, D., Mazurek Melnyk, B., Kuei- Hsiang Hsueh, Jenkins, R., Ding, C. and Durham, J. (2011) Health care in crisis! Can nurse executives' beliefs about and implementation of evidence-based practice be key solutions in health care reform? *Teaching and Learning in Nursing* 6: 73–79

Stabler, S.N., Tejani, A.M., Huynh, F. and Fowkes, C. (2012) Garlic for the prevention of cardiovascular morbidity and mortality in hypertensive patients. *Cochrane Database of Systematic Reviews* Issue 8. Art. No.: CD007653. DOI: 10.1002/14651858.CD007653.pub2. available at http://onlinelibrary.wiley.com/doi/10.1002/14651858.CD007653.pub2/abstract

Standing, M. (ed.) (2005) Perceptions of clinical decision making skills on a developmental journey from student to staff nurse. PhD thesis: University of Kent, Canterbury

Standing, M. (2008) Clinical judgement and decision making in nursing. Nine modes of practice in a revised cognitive continuum. *Journal of Advanced Nursing* 62(1): 124–134

Standing, M. (ed.) (2010) *Clinical Judgement and Decision Making in Nursing and Inter-professional Health Care.* Open University Press: Maidenhead

Stead, L.F., Bergson, G. and Lancaster, T. (2008) Physician advice for smoking cessation. *Cochrane Database of Systematic Reviews,* Issue 2. Art. No.: CD000165. DOI: 10.1002/14651858.CD000165.pub3 available at http://onlinelibrary.wiley.com/doi/10.1002/14651858.CD000165.pub3/abstract

Stillwell, S.B., Fineout-Overholt, E., Melnyk, B.M. and Williamson, K.M. (2010) Asking the clinical question: a key step in evidence based practice. *American Journal of Nursing* 110(3): 58–61

Tabak, R.G., Khoong, E.C., Chambers, D.A. and Brownson, R.C. (2012) Bridging research and practice: models for dissemination and implementation research. *American Journal of Preventive Medicine* 43(3): 337–350

Tanner, C. (2006) Thinking like a nurse: a research-based model of clinical judgement in nursing. *Journal of Nursing Education* 45(6): 204–211

Tebbet, M. and Kennedy, P. (2012) The experience of childbirth for women with spinal cord injuries: an interpretative phenomenological analysis study. *Disability and Rehabilitation* 34(9): 762–769

Theobald, S., Tulloch, O., Crichton, J., Hawkins, K., Zulu, E., Mayaud, P., Parkhurst, J., Whiteside, A. and Standing, H. (2011) Strengthening the research to policy and practice interface: exploring strategies used by research organizations working on sexual and reproductive health and HIV/AIDS. *Health Research Policy and Systems* 9 (Suppl 1): 52 http://www.biomedcentral.com/1478-4505/9/S1/S2

Thompson, C., McCaughan, D., Cullum, N., Sheldon, T. and Raynor, P. (2005) Barriers to evidence-based practice in primary nursing care, why viewing decision making as context is helpful. *Journal of Advanced Nursing* 52(4): 432–444

Thompson, C. and Stapley, S. (2011) Do educational interventions improve nurses' clinical decision making and judgement? A systematic review. *International Journal of Nursing Studies* 48(7): 881–893

Thouless, R.H. and Thouless, C.R. (1953) *Straight and Crooked Thinking*, 4th edn. Hoddder and Stoughton: Sevenoaks

Titler, M.G., Kleiber, C., Steelman, V.J., Rakel, B.A., Budreau, G., Everett, L.Q., Buckwalter, K.C., Tripp-Reimer, T. and Goode, C.J. (2001) The Iowa model of evidence-based practice to promote quality care. *Critical Care Nursing Clinics of North America* 13(4): 497–509

Variend, H. (2012) Capacity confusion (letter). *British Medical Association News* September 1

Wakefield, A.J., Murch, S.H., Anthony, A. and Linnell, J. (1998) Ileal-lymphoid-nodular hyperplasia, non-specific colitis and pervasive developmental disorder in children. *Lancet* 351: 637–641 (paper now withdrawn)

Welsh, B.C. and Farringdon, D.P. (2008) Effect of closed circuit television on crime. *Campbell Collaboration systematic review*. 2 December www.campbellcollaboration.org/lib/download/661/

Wilkinson, J.E., Nutley, S.M. and Davies, H.T.O. (2011) An exploration of the roles of nurse managers in evidence-based practice implementation. *Worldviews on Evidence-Based Nursing* 8(4): 236–246

Wolfe, S.H. and Johnson, R.E. (2005) The break-even point: when medical advances are less important than improving the fidelity with which they are delivered. *Annals of Family Medicine* 3(6): 545–552

Yong, E. (2012) Trials at the ready – preparing for the next pandemic. *British Medical Journal* 344(16): 21–23

Zeitz, K. and McCutcheon, H. (2003) Evidence based practice – to be or not to be that is the question. *International Journal of Nursing Practice* 9(5): 272–279

Appendix: Useful websites

*All accessed in September 2012. All these websites were accurate at the time of going to press. If you are unable to access a link, a simple 'Google' search of the organization should enable you to access the appropriate website. Sites in boxes with ** are considered to be excellent general sites or gateways to other resources.*

AGREE Collaboration (Appraisal of Guidelines for Research and Evaluation) state that 'the potential benefits of practice guidelines are only as good as the quality of the guidelines themselves. To address the variability in practice guideline quality, the AGREE Enterprise was initiated with the development of the original AGREE Instrument'. There is now second version of the instrument: http://www.agreetrust.org/

Bad Science: A website by columnist Ben Goldacre that offers a light-hearted view on health and social care stories from the media and wider: http://www.badscience.net/

Bandolier is a useful and easy to read 'independent journal about evidence-based healthcare', written by Oxford scientists. They offer easy to read overviews of some of the issues and you can browse by topic (http://www.medicine.ox.ac.uk/bandolier/). They also offer a glossary (http://www.medicine.ox.ac.uk/bandolier/glossary.html).

Best Health helps patients and doctors work together by providing them both with the best research evidence about the treatments for many medical conditions: http://besthealth.bmj.com/btuk/home.jsp

---

The Campbell Collaboration helps people make well-informed decisions by preparing, maintaining and disseminating systematic reviews in education, crime and justice, and social welfare: http://www.campbellcollaboration.org/

CASP: Critical Appraisal Skills Programme – the CASP International Network (CASPin) is 'an international collaboration which supports the teaching and learning of critical appraisal skills . . . They have a range of critical appraisal tools: http://www.caspinternational.org/

CEBM: Centre for Evidence Based Medicine aims to 'develop, teach and promote evidence-based healthcare through conferences, workshops and EBM tools so that all healthcare professionals can maintain the highest standards of medicine'. There are online tutorials and critical appraisal tools available: http://www.cebm.net/

CEBMH: Centre for Evidence Based Mental Health aims to 'promote the teaching and practice of evidence-based health care (EBHC) throughout the UK (with special emphasis on evidence-based mental health) and internationally. To develop, evaluate, and disseminate improved methods of using research in practice, and incorporate these in the teaching methods of the CEBMH': http://cebmh.warne.ox.ac.uk/cebmh/index.html

---

The Centre for Reviews and Dissemination (CRD) http://www.york.ac.uk/inst/crd/ is part of the National Institute for Health Research (NIHR) and is a department of the University of York. Their databases and systematic reviews provide research-based information about the effects of important health and social care interventions. To avoid potential conflict of interest, they do not undertake work for or receive funding from the pharmaceutical industry.

They have also produced substantial guidance for professionals actually undertaking systematic reviews (so spreading the word is part of the process of reviewing literature). http://www.york.ac.uk/inst/crd/index_guidance.htm

---

Cochrane Collaboration: Their vision is 'that healthcare decision-making throughout the world will be informed by high-quality, timely research evidence'. They aim to help healthcare providers, policy-makers, patients, their advocates and carers, make well-informed decisions about healthcare, by preparing, updating, and promoting the accessibility of Cochrane Reviews. The reviews are presented as full documents or plain language summaries. The also prepare the largest collection of records of Randomized Controlled Trials in the world, called **CENTRAL, published as part of The Cochrane Library: http://www.cochrane.org/

**Cochrane webliography: This is a great site with links to a wider range of evidence-based practice resources: http://www.cochrane.org/about-us/evidence-based-health-care/webliography

CONSORT (Consolidated Standards of Reporting Trials, 2010) have produced the **CONSORT Statement** available at http://www.consort-statement.org/ which is an evidence-based, minimum set of recommendations for reporting RCTs. It offers a standard way for authors to prepare reports of trial findings, facilitating their complete and transparent reporting, and aiding their critical appraisal and interpretation.

DISCERN: 'Despite a rapid growth in the provision of consumer health information, the quality of the information remains variable. DISCERN is a brief questionnaire which provides users with a valid and reliable way of assessing the quality of written information on treatment choices for a health problem. DISCERN can also be used by authors and publishers of information on treatment choices as a guide to the standard which users are entitled to expect': http://www.discern.org.uk/

DOH: Department of Health including Public Health, Adult Social Care, and the NHS. This site provides links to national guidance, benchmarking standards and policy: http://www.dh.gov.uk/en/index.htm

EMPHO offers an Introduction to **Evidence-Informed Public Health** and a **Compendium of Critical Appraisal Tools for Public Health Practice** available at: http://www.empho.org.uk/Download/Public/11615/1/CA%20Tools%20 for%20Public%20Health.pdf

Essence of Care: The benchmarking process outlined in 'Essence of Care' (Department of Health 2010) aims to help practitioners to share and compare practice, enabling them to adopt a structured approach to identifying the best practice and to develop action plans to remedy poor practice. It contains 12 benchmarks, and aims to support localized quality improvement available at: http://www.dh.gov.uk/en/Publicationsandstatistics/Publications/Publication-sPolicyAndGuidance/DH_119969

Evidence in Health and Social Care: this site is a comprehensive and excellent gateway to other sites, standards and guidance. You can search by topic, link to NICE guidelines etc. (http://www.evidence.nhs.uk/) and there is a specific **public health section: http://www.evidence.nhs.uk/nhs-evidence-content/public-health

It also provide links to a range of other sources such as **topic specific updates:** http://www.evidence.nhs.uk/nhs-evidence-content/evidence-updates

---

Evidence Updates highlight new evidence relating to published accredited guidance. They do not replace current guidance and do not provide formal

practice recommendations. It is organized by topic: http://www.evidence.nhs.
uk/nhs-evidence-content/evidence-updates

GOOGLE SCHOLAR: This site is 'one better' than Google or a general search
engine. You can search for topics but also put dates in and it generally provides more academic sources. There are sometimes direct links to the papers:
http://scholar.google.co.uk/

HSCP: Health and Care Professions Council. Their role is to protect the public
as a regulatory body for: arts therapists, biomedical scientists, chiropodists/
podiatrists, clinical scientists, dieticians, hearing aid dispensers, occupational
therapists, operating department practitioners, orthoptists, paramedics, physiotherapists, practitioner psychologists, prosthetists/orthotists, radiographers,
social workers in England and speech and language therapists: http://www.
hpc-uk.org/

Health Knowledge: 'This online learning resource is for anyone working in
health, social care and well-being across the NHS, local authorities, the voluntary, and the private sector. The resource allows you to access a broad range of
learning materials for personal use or for teaching purposes in order to help
everyone expand their public health knowledge': http://www.healthknowl-
edge.org.uk/

Institute of Health and Wellbeing: This site offers a variety of critical appraisal
checklists from Glasgow University: http://www.gla.ac.uk/researchinstitutes/
healthwellbeing/research/generalpractice/ebp/checklists/#d.en.19536

King's Fund: The King's Fund seeks to understand how the health system in
England can be improved. Using that insight, they work with individuals and
organizations to shape policy, transform services and bring about behaviour
change: http://www.kingsfund.org.uk/

Map of medicine health guides shows the ideal, evidence-based patient
journey for common and important conditions. It claims to be a high-level
overview to be used by professionals that can be shared with patients: http://
healthguides.mapofmedicine.com/choices/map/index.html

National Guideline Clearinghouse is a public resource for evidence-based
clinical practice guidelines: http://www.guideline.gov/

Netting the Evidence is now a specific search engine for all things related to
evidence based practice: http://tinyurl.com/2poh3a

NISCHR: The National Institute for Social Care and Health Research
(http://www.wales.nhs.uk/sites3/home.cfm?orgid=952). This is the Welsh

Government body that works with others to develop strategy and policy for research in the NHS and social care in Wales. It does this by:

• Streamlining Research
• Supporting Excellence And Innovation
• Investing In The Future

NSFs (National Service Frameworks): This site offers strategies for cancer, Chronic Heart Disease, Chronic Obstructive Pulmonary Disease, Diabetes, Kidney Care, Long Term Conditions, Mental Health, Older People and Stroke: http://www.nhs.uk/NHSEngland/NSF/Pages/Nationalserviceframeworks.aspx

NHS CHOICES: This site offers an A–Z of common conditions, a health encyclopaedia and an A–Z of medicines and symptom checker: http://www.nhs.uk/Pages/HomePage.aspx

---

**NICE National Institute for Health and Clinical Excellence (NICE) is an independent organization responsible for providing national guidance on promoting good health and preventing and treating ill health (http://www.nice.org.uk/). The guidelines can be searched and are grouped under:

• conditions and treatments
• procedures and devices
• public health

There are also **NICE quality standards** (http://www.nice.org.uk/aboutnice/qualitystandards/qualitystandards.jsp). NICE quality standards are said to be 'central to supporting the Government's vision for an NHS and Social Care system focussed on delivering the best possible outcomes for people who use services, as detailed in the Health and Social Care Act (2012)' (http://www.legislation.gov.uk/ukpga/2012/7/enacted). There are some quality standards for social work in development too.

NICE Pathways provides 'quick and easy access, topic by topic, to the range of guidance published by NICE, including quality standards, technology appraisals, clinical and public health guidance and NICE implementation tools'. They assert that pathways are simple to navigate and allow users to explore in increasing detail NICE recommendations and advice, giving the user confidence that they are up to date: http://pathways.nice.org.uk/

NMC: Nursing and Midwifery Council (NMC) the regulatory body for nurses and midwives. They also offer some standards and guidance: http://www.nmc-uk.org/

PRODIGY: This contains a number of resources to support clinicians working in general practice and is a reliable source of evidence-based information and practical 'know how' about the common conditions managed in primary care. PRODIGY is aimed at healthcare professionals working in primary and first-contact care: http://prodigy.clarity.co.uk/home

Research Mindedness in Social work: Although this site is no longer being updated the glossary is still relevant: http://www.resmind.swap.ac.uk/content/00_other/glossary.htm

---

SCIE: The Social Care Institute for Excellence (http://www.scie.org.uk/) aims to gather, analyse, share knowledge about what works and translate that knowledge into practical resources, learning materials and services including training and consultancy. The notion of **co-production is fundamental to what they do and this is where SCIE aims to co-produce their work with people who use services and carers. They have developed a set of principles and a strategy to support this idea. They produce:

- A comprehensive, searchable **database** of information: Social Care Online http://www.scie-socialcareonline.org.uk/default.asp
- **Briefings** on developing research http://www.scie.org.uk/publications/briefings/index.asp
- A database of **good practice examples** http://www.scie.org.uk/goodpractice/browse/default.aspx

As well as these there are some more **general information sources**

- **Practical guides** on major issues in social care and social work http://www.scie.org.uk/publications/guides/index.asp
- **At-a-glance summaries** http://www.scie.org.uk/publications/ataglance/index.asp
- **eLearning resources** such as teaching guides on such topics as personalization and dementia http://www.scie.org.uk/publications/elearning/index.asp
- **Social Care TV channel** which includes a collection of video resources http://www.scie.org.uk/socialcaretv/index.asp

---

SIGN: The Scottish Intercollegiate Guidelines Network which brings together evidence-based guidelines has a range of appraisal checklists: http://sign.ac.uk/methodology/checklists.html

TRIP: Turning Research Into Practice (TRIP) Database. The TRIP Database provides direct, hyperlinked access to a large collection of evidence-based material on the web, as well as articles from online journals. Needs log in but is free: http://www.tripdatabase.com/

The **What is . . .? series** is intended to demystify some of the terminology, techniques and practices used to assess clinical and economic evidence within healthcare: http://www.whatisseries.co.uk/whatis/

Index

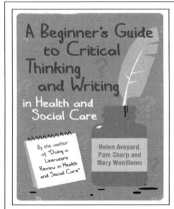

A BEGINNER'S GUIDE TO CRITICAL THINKING AND WRITING IN HEALTH AND SOCIAL CARE

Helen Aveyard, Pam Sharp and Mary Woolliams

9780335243662 (Paperback)
August 2011

eBook also available

Ever wondered what critical thinking is and how you can do it?

Ever struggled to write a critical essay?

Then this is the book for you. This is a beginner's guide to the skills of critical thinking, critical writing and critical appraisal in health and social care, and talks you through every stage of becoming a critical thinker. Each chapter tackles a different aspect of the process and using examples and simple language shows you how it's done. An essential purchase for students and qualified healthcare staff alike.

www.openup.co.uk

OPEN UNIVERSITY PRESS
McGraw - Hill Education

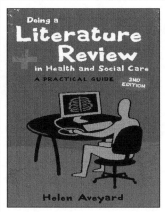

DOING A LITERATURE REVIEW IN HEALTH AND SOCIAL CARE
A Practical Guide
Second Edition

Helen Aveyard

9780335238859 (Paperback)
2010

eBook also available

This bestselling book is a step-by-step guide to doing a literature review in health and social care. It is vital reading for all those undertaking their undergraduate or postgraduate dissertation or any research module which involves a literature review.

The new edition has been fully updated and provides a practical guide to the different types of literature that you may be encountered when undertaking a literature review.

Key features:

- Includes examples of commonly occurring real life scenarios encountered by students
- Provides advice on how to follow a clearly defined search strategy
- Details a wide range of critical appraisal tools that can be utilised

www.openup.co.uk

OPEN UNIVERSITY PRESS
McGraw · Hill Education

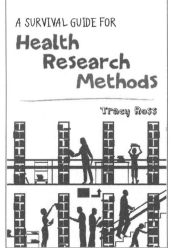

A SURVIVAL GUIDE FOR HEALTH RESEARCH METHODS

Tracy Ross

9780335244737 (Paperback)
2012

eBook also available

This handy book is an ideal companion for all health and nursing students looking for an accessible guide to research. Written in a friendly style, the book takes the stress out of research learning by offering realistic, practical guidance and demystifying research methods jargon.

Key features:

- A great first book for students and practitioners new to the subject.
- Packed with examples and case studies that highlights good and bad practice in research
- Jargon free

OPEN UNIVERSITY PRESS
McGraw - Hill Education

www.openup.co.uk